Ergebnisse der Anatomie und Entwicklungsgeschichte
Advances in Anatomy, Embryology and Cell Biology
Revues d'anatomie et de morphologie expérimentale

Springer-Verlag Berlin Heidelberg New York

This journal publishes reviews and critical articles covering the entire field of normal anatomy (cytology, histology, cyto- and histochemistry, electron microscopy, macroscopy, experimental morphology and embryology and comparative anatomy). Papers dealing with anthropology and clinical morphology will also be accepted with the aim of encouraging co-operation between anatomy and related disciplines.

Papers, which may be in English, French or German, are normally commissioned, but original papers and communications may be submitted and will be considered so long as they deal with a subject comprehensively and meet the requirements of the Ergebnisse.

For speed of publication and breadth of distribution, this journal appears in single issues which can be purchased separately; 6 issues constitute one volume.

It is a fundamental condition that manuscripts submitted should not have been published elsewhere, in this or any other country, and the author must undertake not to publish elsewhere at a later date.

25 copies of each paper are supplied free of charge.

Les résultats publient des sommaires et des articles critiques concernant l'ensemble du domaine de l'anatomie normale (cytologie, histologie, cyto et histochimie, microscopie électronique, macroscopie, morphologie expérimentale, embryologie et anatomie comparée. Seront publiés en outre les articles traitant de l'anthropologie et de la morphologie clinique, en vue d'encourager la collaboration entre l'anatomie et les disciplines voisines.

Seront publiés en priorité les articles expressément demandés nous tiendrons toutefois compte des articles qui nous seront envoyés dans la mesure où ils traitent d'un sujet dans son ensemble et correspondent aux standards des «Résultats». Les publications seront faites en langues anglaise, allemande et française.

Dans l'intérêt d'une publication rapide et d'une large diffusion les travaux publiés paraitront dans des cahiers individuels, diffusés séparément: 6 cahiers forment un volume.

En principe, seuls les manuscrits qui n'ont encore été publiés ni dans le pays d'origine ni à l'étranger peuvent nous être soumis. L'auteur d'engage en outre à ne pas les publier ailleurs ultérieurement.

Les auteurs recevront 25 exemplaires gratuits de leur publication.

Die Ergebnisse dienen der Veröffentlichung zusammenfassender und kritischer Artikel aus dem Gesamtgebiet der normalen Anatomie (Cytologie, Histologie, Cyto- und Histochemie, Elektronenmikroskopie, Makroskopie, experimentelle Morphologie und Embryologie und vergleichende Anatomie). Aufgenommen werden ferner Arbeiten anthropologischen und morphologisch-klinischen Inhaltes, mit dem Ziel die Zusammenarbeit zwischen Anatomie und Nachbardisziplinen zu fördern.

Zur Veröffentlichung gelangen in erster Linie angeforderte Manuskripte, jedoch werden auch eingesandte Arbeiten und Originalmitteilungen berücksichtigt, sofern sie ein Gebiet umfassend abhandeln und den Anforderungen der „Ergebnisse" genügen. Die Veröffentlichungen erfolgen in englischer, deutscher oder französischer Sprache.

Die Arbeiten erscheinen im Interesse einer raschen Veröffentlichung und einer weiten Verbreitung als einzeln berechnete Hefte; je 6 Hefte bilden einen Band.

Grundsätzlich dürfen nur Manuskripte eingesandt werden, die vorher weder im Inland noch im Ausland veröffentlicht worden sind. Der Autor verpflichtet sich, sie auch nachträglich nicht an anderen Stellen zu publizieren.

Die Mitarbeiter erhalten von ihren Arbeiten zusammen 25 Freiexemplare.

Manuscripts should be addressed to/Envoyer les manuscrits à/Manuskripte sind zu senden an:

Prof. Dr. A. BRODAL, Universitetet i Oslo, Anatomisk Institutt, Karl Johans Gate 47 (Domus Media), Oslo 1/Norwegen

Prof. W. HILD, Department of Anatomy, The University of Texas Medical Branch, Galveston, Texas 77550 (USA).

Prof. Dr. R. ORTMANN, Anatomisches Institut der Universität, D-5000 Köln-Lindenthal, Lindenburg.

Prof. Dr. T. H. SCHIEBLER, Anatomisches Institut der Universität, Koellikerstraße 6, D-8700 Würzburg

Prof. Dr. G. TÖNDURY, Direktion der Anatomie, Gloriastraße 19, CH-8006 Zürich.

Prof. Dr. E. WOLFF, Collège de France, Laboratoire d'Embryologie Expérimentale, 49 bis Avenue de la belle Gabrielle, Nogent-sur-Marne 49/France.

Ergebnisse der Anatomie und Entwicklungsgeschichte
Advances in Anatomy, Embryology and Cell Biology
Revues d'anatomie et de morphologie expérimentale

45·6

Editores
A. Brodal, Oslo · W. Hild, Galveston · R. Ortmann, Köln
T. H. Schiebler, Würzburg · G. Töndury, Zürich · E. Wolff, Paris

Hans-Rainer Duncker

The Lung Air Sac System of Birds

A contribution to the functional anatomy of the respiratory apparatus

With 41 Figures

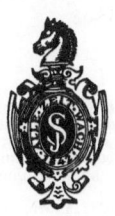

Springer-Verlag Berlin Heidelberg GmbH 1971

Prof. Dr. Dr. H.-R. Duncker
Department of Anatomy
University of Gießen, Germany
D-63 Gießen, Friedrichstraße 24

.

Habilitationsschrift, presented to and accepted by the Medical Faculty of the University of Hamburg on November 5th, 1968

The Carl Christiansen Gedächtnis-Preis Hamburg 1969 has been awarded for this thesis

ISBN 978-3-540-05659-1   ISBN 978-3-662-10354-8 (eBook)
DOI 10.1007/978-3-662-10354-8

Dedicated to

Prof. Dr. Dr. E. Horstmann

in cordial gratitude and admiration

Contents

Review of Literature

Starting with the first observations of Coiter (1573) up to the physiologic studies of today (Piiper, Pfeifer, and Scheid, 1969; Piiper, Drees, and Scheid, 1970; Scheid and Piiper, 1969, 1970) the manyfold efforts to understand the structure and function of the avian lung intersperse the history of comparative anatomy and physiology. Even today this discussion has not conclusively been settled. King (1957) emphasizes the "remarkable fact that after three centuries of research all the great questions of the functional anatomy of the avian respiratory tract still remain unanswered. It could well be that one reason has been the failure to recognize in time the fundamental variation in structure and function of the respiratory tract in the different avian species". Fisher, in 1955, writes: „Without knowledge of the detailed structure, the manner in which the system functions will remain hypothetical". With this quotation King (1966) ends the introduction of the most recent survey, that also was not able to conclusively solve the important anatomical and functional problems.

Since Coiter (1573), Fabricius ab Aquapendente (1615) and Harvey (1651) described the openings on the ventral surface of the avian lung, and their connections with the air sacs, and also investigated the respiratory mechanism of birds, the lung air sac system of birds has been studied by many comparative anatomists and physiologists. The extension of the air sac system between the musculature of the extremities and as far as into the bones has first been described by Camper (1774, 1776) and Hunter (1774). After Fuld's (1816) description of the parabronchi, Geoffroy-Saint-Hilaire's (1818) of the ventrobronchi and Colas' (1825) of the dorsobronchi, Retzius (1832) emphasizes the special structure of the avian lung in its deviation from the mammalian lung. In the course of his report he points out that no blindly ending bronchial tree exists but that the superficial bronchi are connected to each other via parabronchi, and thus that each passage leads back to the primary bronchus.

A vast amount of specific data is described in the many following, mostly short reports. They always refer to one or very few species and moreover are limited to parts of the lung air sac system with the systematically important syrinx getting most of the attention and treatment. These older studies, which Campana (1875) and Fischer (1905) have best compiled, do not give an adequate concept of the structure of the avian respiratory apparatus, since most of the data are too cursory and not reliably exact. That is also true for often quoted studies as those of Owen (1830, 1835a, b), Weber (1842), Schulze (1871), Huxley (1882), Parker (1883) and Beddard (1885, 1886a, b, 1888, 1896, 1898). Moreover, not only many misinterpretations but numerous false observations are contained in these works as is shown by the very exact synopses of Gadow (1891) and Oppel (1905) which themselves are full of contradictions.

The works of Sappey (1847) and of Campana (1875) are especially important parts of the old literature. Sappey gives a very exact, well illustrated account

of the lungs and air sacs of a duck. Campana describes in a very detailed manner
the lung with its bronchial system and the air sacs as far as the last diverticula
in a chicken. Besides, the studies of Strasser (1877) and Roché (1891) are of
certain importance, since they demonstrate the extension of the air sacs in a
number of species on a broad comparative basis. Just as these monographs,
the compiling articles of textbooks and handbooks of the last century (Cuvier,
1810; Stannius, 1846; Owen, 1866; Gadow, 1891; Gegenbaur, 1901) discuss the
concepts of the functions of the lung air sac system. This discussion is especially
integrated into the works of Baer (1896), Soum (1896) and Siefert (1896), the
first, more extensive, physiologic works about the avian respiration which,
however, contain an abundance of misinterpretations.

The anatomical literature about the avian lung and the respiratory apparatus
is not so extensive in our century. After Rainey's (1849) description of the cross
linking of the finest air passages, Fischer (1905), in a remarkable study, shows
conclusive proof of the air capillaries and describes their arrangement and systematic changes; less careful is his demonstration of the bronchial system. In 1908
Müller gives a detailed description of the pigeon air sacs. Schulze (1908) studies
the lungs of the African ostrich according to their external appearance and also
discusses the function of the air sacs (Schulze, 1909, 1912). The term "bronchi
recurrentes" for the saccobronchi which was supposed to give a functional interpretation of not only these structures, but also of the general lung structure,
dates back to a very short note of Schulze (1910). Juillet (1911a, c, 1912a, b)
demonstrates the bronchial system to a certain extent and also considers the
deviation in a number of species from different families, using illustrations of
good quality. Zimmer (1935) presents a very good analysis of the locomotor
system of birds, emphasizing the reciprocal independence of wing and respiratory
motions and for the first time satisfactorily interpreting the function of the
processus uncinati of the avian ribs.

Stanislaus (1937) investigates the hummingbird lung and demonstrates its
bronchial system. Vos (1937) recognizes the lack of the so-called recurrent bronchi
in penguins. Gilbert (1939) again demonstrates the pigeon air sac system and
Richardson (1939) describes and discusses the subcutaneous air sacs of a pelican.
Gier (1952) reports development and position of the air sacs of a loon. Akester
(1960), using injection preparations, thoroughly describes the bronchial system
in three species of poultry, Mennega and Calhoun (1968) demonstrate the respiratory system of the duck and Wetherbee (1951) precisely describes the air sacs
of the house sparrow. King and Atherton (1970) compare the air sacs of the
turkey with those of domestic fowl. Duncker (1970b) demonstrates the topographical relations of the lungs and the air sac system and their systematical
deviation. Also the topography of the abdominal air sacs is clarified which, since
Huxley's (1882) report on the kiwi air sacs, had usually been described falsely
for the rest of the birds in the literature of the following decades.

Krause (1922), Bremer (1939), Cover (1953a, b), King (1956) and Rigdon
(1959) above all report the microscopic anatomy of the avian lung in single
species of domestic birds. Duncker (1969) demonstrates the deviation of the parabronchial structure, starting with penguins up to song birds. Moreover the
ultrastructure of air capillaries has been extensively studied in chickens, pigeons

and geese (de Groodt, Sebruyns and Lagasse, 1960; Bargmann and Knoop, 1961; Policard, Collet, and Martin, 1962; Tyler and Pangborn, 1964; Petrik, 1967; Petrik and Riedel, 1968a, b; Lambson and Cohn, 1968; Akester, 1970; MacDonald, 1970). Conclusive evidence for an uninterrupted lining of the air capillaries with an extremely thin epithelium that is always covered by a two-layered osmiophilic film, was given in these studies. In a number of recent works also the structure and ultrastructure of other elements of the parabronchi, the epithelial cells outside the air capillaries, the elastic fibers and the muscle cells and their innervation as well as the nerves and a receptor complex are demonstrated (Akester and Mann, 1969; Cook and King, 1969a, b, 1970; Cowie and King, 1969; King, Ellis, and Watts, 1967; King and Cowie, 1968, 1969; McLelland, 1969).

Developmental studies have been performed mainly on chickens. They pursue the development of the lung and the air sacs. The first such study is by Rathke (1828). Selenka (1866) has especially pursued the development of the air sacs and Larsell (1914) and Locy and Larsell (1916a, b) provide a very detailed study of the development of the bronchial system and the air sacs. Bertelli (1905) and Poole (1909) study the development of the septa and their relations to the air sac development. Delphia (1958) describes the air sac development in a duck and very clearly the development of the secondary bronchi in the sparrow (Delphia, 1961). Individual embryological observations on chicken embryos are described by Juillet (1911b), Daniel (1957) and Petrik (1967). Daniel gives supplementing data on a song bird. Romanoff (1960) compiles the knowledge about the ontogeny of the lung and the air sacs.

Up to date, only the poultry is anatomically and especially physiologically well studied. Many individual data are indeed known through these studies, the basic principle of the respiratory system of birds, however, remained obscure both in anatomical and in physiological respects. This is very expressively stated in articles of text- and handbooks and reviews of Stresemann (1927–1934), Groebbels (1932), Marcus (1937), Grau (1943), Portmann (1950b), Fisher (1955), Goodrich (1958), Stolpe and Zimmer (1959), Salt and Zeuthen (1960), Diesselhorst (1964) and King (1966).

The history of the investigation of the lung air sac system of the birds is a sequence of false suppositions, unreliable interpretations, and fundamental mistakes. The transfer of data of the structure and function of the mammalian respiratory system on the avian respiratory system, without any reflective criticism, led to the confusion indicated. The historical assumptions are reduced only stepwise and hesitantly, usually forced by new anatomical findings. Besides the inadequate anatomical data, the difficulty to perform physiological experiments during the last century, led to an abundance of hypotheses, the majority of which could not be proved, however. As one of the last absurd effects of such phantastic hypotheses appears the work of Thilo (1915) "The air sacs of birds as blocking mechanism" by which the wings were supposed to be kept in extended position. Today this vast number of hypotheses and ideas has only a scientific-historical meaning.

At the end of the last century the differentiation of the avian respiratory apparatus into a rigid gas exchanging portion, the lung with the parabronchi, and a ventilating portion, the air sac system connected to the primary bronchus, was still not completely understood. This is shown by the theme of a competition, which was studied by Baer (1896): "About the respiratory function of the air sacs". It is true that Baer assigned the air sacs a bellows function, however, at the same time he assumes that the movements of the thorax during flight are regulated "naturally", "since the thorax must be fixed for the action of the originating flight musculature" and that the lung ventilation is performed by the massage of the axillary air sacs. This concept can be found throughout even the most recent literature (Buddenbrock, 1928; Herzog, 1968).

The assumption that the lung ventilation is caused by a marked volume change of the lung is found in the works of Soum (1896), Victorow (1909), Schulze (1912), Buddenbrock (1928) and Makowski (1938a, b). Even Salt and Zeuthen (1960) still report this viewpoint, even though Sappey had already in 1847 assured the general immobility of the lung. In the following years, however, the bellows theory for the function of the air sacs was accepted by most authors.

The concept of an antagonistic function of the anterior and posterior air sacs, which for the first time was published by Perrault (1676), is also advocated by Sappey (1847). Experiments on the opened abdominal cavity had shown that during inspiration the abdominal air sacs collapse, while the anterior air sacs are filled, and that this process is reversed during expiration. This observation can be made only by opening the abdomen since the flow resistance out of the abdominal into the anterior air sacs via the lung is smaller than the resistance in the course of filling all air sacs via the trachea. This concept too is held up to the middle of this century. Most persistently this antagonism for the transportation of respiratory air through the lung is maintained for the diving of birds (Bethe, 1925; Marcus, 1937). The works of Scholander (1940) and others, which were compiled by Andersen (1966) have for the first time shown that the respiration of birds similar to other vertebrates stops during diving. This concept was confirmed for the domestic goose by Cohn, Krog and Shannon (1968).

The majority of investigators after 1925 advocate the bellows theory with synchronous action of the anterior and posterior air sacs, supported by a number of distinct experimental results, which were compiled by Scharnke (1934). The point of controversy which remained unsolved was the passage of the respiratory air through the lung parenchyma. This is not surprising considering the state of the anatomical knowledge which, for lung structure, had been obtained from only a small number of poultry. By the works of Strasser (1877) and Roché (1891) the variety of the air sacs, dependent on the multiplicity of bird species, had become partly known. Juillet (1912a) studied the bronchial system of 21 species which, however, caused by his selection of the species, proved to be only variations of one type of bronchial system. Neither Stanislaus (exact description of the hummingbird lung 1937) nor Vos (lack of recurrent bronchi in penguins 1937) pursue the obvious conclusions that arise from their findings. King (1966), in a very careful synopsis, compiled all data about the lung and air sac structure, as well as the known physiologic data, without being able, however, to emphasize a principle of structure that could have stimulated the physiological research. Duncker (1968a, 1970a) demonstrated the deviations in the structure of the bronchial system and of the connections of the air sacs appearing in the class of birds, according to systematic points of view, and drew the resulting functional conclusions.

The investigation of the avian respiration was performed almost completely on particular species of poultry. Above all, generally only the respiration at rest of the experimental animals was measured and not seldom even in supine position of the animals (Baer, 1896; Soum, 1896; Victorow, 1909; Cohn and Shannon, 1968). The very complex structure of the intrapulmonal bronchial system of these animals, which so far had not been sufficiently understood, made it impossible to faultlessly interpret the physiological experimental results. In the supine position, the mobil intestinal tract moves dorsally and closes the entrances into the two abdominal air sacs so that they cannot contribute to the ventilation and therefore the lung ventilation is heavily disturbed. Thus, conclusions relating to the normal respiration cannot be drawn from these experiments. Resulting from the ignorance of these contexts the interpretation of findings has often been useless or false, even though the studies contain an abundance of exact data that could have excellently been interpreted with the use of correct anatomical knowledge. This is true for the physiological works of Baer (1896) and Soum (1896) via Scharnke (1938) up to Cohn and Shannon (1968).

In order to interpret the unclear experimental results, structures were postulated that were not present anatomically and were never proved, as sphincter apparatuses or valves in primary and secondary bronchi (Brandes, 1923, 1924; Bethe, 1925; Portier, 1928; Dotterweich, 1930a, b; Vos, 1935, 1937). The sphincters of smooth muscle at the ostia of primary, secondary and saccobronchi into the air sacs were also found in the literature for a long time (Eberth, 1863; Fischer, 1905; Schulze, 1910). However they contain only portions of the circular musculature of the primary and secondary bronchi and they were interpreted as totally closing muscle rings because of false observations. This concept was rejected a few years later (Scharnke, 1934; Dotterweich, 1936; Scharnke, 1938), but a satisfactory explanation could still not be provided as is also shown in the synopses (Zeuthen, 1942; Salt and Zeuthen, 1960; Sturkie, 1965; King, 1966) which in this respect do not differ from earlier handbook articles (Babak, 1921; Bethe, 1925; Scharnke, 1934).

Hazelhoff (1943, in English 1951) in an excellent study attains an uniform interpretation of the experimental data, basing on knowledge of the anatomy of the bronchial system that by far exceeds the contemporary studies. Following concepts of earlier investigators he develops a theory of a completely flow dynamical regulation of the avian lung respiration which is based on the structure and position of the bronchi. However, it must be mentioned that already in 1936 Dotterweich basing on correct observations had conceived this theory in its main components. He was not able to fully prove this theory by anatomical and physico-physiological findings, though. One of the few studies following Hazelhoff's (Biggs and King, 1957), essentially proves the theory of Hazelhoff, while the work of Shepard, Sladen, Peterson, and Enns (1959) does not lead to any new concepts or data. The compiling studies of Salt and Zeuthen (1960) and Sturkie (1965) very critically report the work of Hazelhoff. The reason for this criticism must be sought in the fact that up to date no comparative anatomical study has been made, which precisely demonstrates the different parts of the lung-air sac system in their structure and connections, and which provides a satisfactory amount of comparative material in order to discuss the theory of Hazelhoff, to differentiate, and to stimulate new physiological investigations.

Resulting Problems

Resulting from this situation following problems arise for the study presented:

Regarding the vast amount of existing but partly contradictory findings it becomes necessary to study again the total system of the avian lung and air sacs in a large number of species, without undertaking the task to sift and compile all data dispersed in the literature with their many faults. This only would cause the study to swell in volume but not in clarity. During a revision of the literature one is strikingly puzzled that important relations and facts have been considered only incompletely and usually have been reported incorrectly.

The species investigated are supposed to include the variety of the birds according to systematic position, type of function and body size. But the study is totally dedicated to the problem of the respiratory apparatus, omitting those parts of the air sac system which are known to pneumatise parts of the skeleton as the lightest structural element of the avian body (Duncker, 1968b). Also the air sac diverticula that are situated between the different organs and bones as well as around joints and muscle origins having other functions, are not demonstrated. Also the problems of the comparative anatomy of the individual findings is not supposed to be discussed in this study, this will be left to future publications. By comparing the individual structure elements throughout the whole class of birds the functionally important parts of the respiratory apparatus are to be worked out and thus the changes that have affected the respiratory apparatus according to the systematic position, the type of function and the size of the individual species are to be made recognizable. While bronchial system and air sacs are exactly demonstrated, the vessel system of the lung is only cursorily treated.

It will be shown that the avian trunk has motion systems for wing and leg movements, and for respiratory motions, that are independent of each other, both in flying and running and in swimming and diving birds. The nine air sacs usually present, one impar and four paired, are to be arranged into the group of the five anterior air sacs that are of lesser importance to the lung ventilation, and the group of the two posterior air sac pairs that, functioning as bellows, ventilate the lung. The lung is extended as a system of mostly rigid tubes. According to the concept of Hazelhoff, that is heavily supported by the results of these anatomical studies, the bronchial system of the avian lung is continually perfused in one direction during inspiration and expiration. This is true for that portion of the lung which is present in all birds as the "paleopulmo" and which occupies the larger part of or the whole lung.

In the species systematically higher, the "neopulmo" is added which, at the beginning, is very small and with ascending development towards the song birds occupies the laterocaudal part of the lung. It probably is used for the slight respiration at rest. This differentiation has very probably effected the phylogenetic development since it has created the physiological basis for the development of the variably adapted small and smallest birds.

Besides, it can be shown that the development of this respiratory system in the course of phylogeny is connected to the special type of embryonal development within the egg which by its air space makes possible an air respiration a few days before hatching and thus allows the development of a first net of air capillaries of lung parabronchi before their functional use. Air capillaries with their minute diameter and a resulting high surface tension at the tissue air border cannot be unfolded by muscular forces after collapsing as can the alveoles of a mammalian lung. Resulting from this physical structural peculiarity it becomes intelligible that air capillaries are existent only as rigid tubes in a volume constant lung, and also that they cannot be unfolded under birth but must be developed before hatching, utilizing air respiration, when the gas exchange is still performed by the chorioallantois. Finally, the peculiar characteristics of structure and function of the avian lung are compared to those of the mammalian lung.

I am greatly indebted to Prof. Dr. Dr. E. Horstmann for the constant sponsorship of this investigation, the critical discussion of this publication and the guidance of this work as Habilitationsschrift.

Material and Methods

Systematic and topography of the bronchial system and the air sacs as well as their connections were studied by means of injection preparations. The method developed for the production of these preparations has been extensively described (Duncker, Haufe, and Schlüter, 1964; Duncker and Schlüter, 1964). After evacuation of the lung air sac system mostly silicone rubber was injected, more seldom latex milk or an acryl resin. Birds that had very recently died, could very well be used for the injection, enabling the author to study experimental material that was systematically wide spread.

For the donation of dead animals I am gratefully indebted to the following persons and institutions:

Tierpark Carl Hagenbeck, Hamburg-Stellingen; Dr. R. Faust, Zoologischer Garten der Stadt Frankfurt am Main; „Schwanenvater" Harald Nieß, Hamburg-Billstedt; „Storchen-vater" Wilhelm Schwen, Hamburg-Langenhorn; Tierheim Süderstraße des Hamburger Tierschutzvereins von 1814 e.V., and Zoologische Handlung Hans-Rudolf Dannehl, Hamburg 20. Moreover, I am appreciative to many persons for the donation of dead birds who cannot all be named at this point.

With the assistance of a financial support of the Joachim Jungius-Gesellschaft der Wissenschaften e.V., Hamburg, I was able to travel to Cornwall/England in the spring of 1967. There I had the possibility to study birds unobtainable in Germany, which died during the Torrey Canyon catastrophe. For their assistance in procuring the material I wish to express my appreciation especially to Superintendent J. Kerr, London and Chief-Inspector R. Gardener, Truro/Cornwall of the Royal Society for the Prevention of Cruelty to Animals, as well as Dr. C. J. F. Coombs, Truro/Cornwall. Grateful acknowledgements are made to Dr. Ch. Perrins of the Edward Grey Institute of Field Ornithology, Oxford, Dr. G. G. Dunnet, Culterty Field Station Newburgh of the University of Aberdeen and Chief Warden P. Wormell, The Nature Conservancy, Isle of Rhum, Inverness-Shire for the procurement of specimens of rare species.

Following species were studied:

Spheniscidae, Penguins
  *King Penguin, *Aptenodytes patagonica* J.F. Miller

*Rockhopper Penguin, *Eudyptes cristatus* (J. F. Miller)
Gentoo Penguin, *Pygoscelis papua* (Forster)
Magellanic Penguin, *Spheniscus magellanicus* (Forster) (1 specimen)
Black-footed Penguin, *Spheniscus demersus* (L.) (1 specimen)
Dromiceiidae, Emus
Emu, *Dromiceius novaehollandiae* (Latham)
Rheidae, Rheas
*American Rhea, *Rhea americana* (L.)
Darwin's Rhea, *Pterocnemia pennata* (d'Orbigny)
Phalacrocoracidae, Cormorants
*Green Cormorant, *Phalacrocorax aristotelis* (L.)
Sulidae, Boobies and Gannets
Northern Gannet, *Sula bassana* (L.)
Masked Booby, *Sula dactylatra* Lesson (1 specimen)
Procellariidae, Procellariids
*Manx Shearwater, *Puffinus puffinus* (Brünnich)
*Arctic Fulmar, *Fulmarus glacialis* (L.)
Hydrobatidae, Storm Petrels
Leach's Petrel, *Oceanodroma leucorrhoa* (Vieillot) (1 specimen)
Storm Petrel, *Hydrobates pelagicus* (L.) (1 specimen)
Gaviidae, Loons
*Black-throated Diver, *Gavia arctica* (L.)
Great Northern Diver, *Gavia immer* (Brünnich) (1 specimen)
Podicipedidae, Grebes
Great Crested Grebe, *Podiceps cristatus* (L.)
Little Grebe, *Podiceps ruficollis* (Pallas)
Ardeidae, Herons
*Grey Heron, *Ardea cinerea* (L.)
Night Heron, *Nycticorax nycticorax* (L.)
Ciconiidae, Storks
*White Stork, *Ciconia ciconia* L.
Seddle Bill, *Ephippiorhynchus senegalensis* (Shaw) (1 specimen)
Phoenicopteridae, Flamingoes
Greater Flamingo, *Phoenicopterus ruber* L.
Anatidae, Swans, Geese, Ducks and Mergansers
*Mute Swan, *Cygnus olor* (Gmelin)
Whooper Swan, *Cygnus cygnus* (L.)
*Black Swan, *Cygnus atratus* (Latham)
Greylag Goose, *Anser anser* (L.)
*Common Shelduck, *Tadorna tadorna* (L.)
Mandarin Duck, *Aix galericulata* (L.)
European Wigeon, *Anas penelope* L.
*Teal, *Anas crecca* L.
*Northern Mallard, *Anas platyrhynchos* L.
European Pochard, *Aythya ferina* (L.)
*Tufted Duck, *Aythya fuligula* (L.)
Common Eider, *Somateria mollissima* (L.)
Black Scoter, *Melanitta nigra* (L.)
Velvet Scoter, *Melanitta fusca* (L.)
Common Goldeneye, *Bucephala clangula* (L.)
Smew, *Mergus albellus* L.
Goosander, *Mergus merganser* L.
Accipitridae, Diurnal Birds of Prey
*Common Buzzard, *Buteo buteo* (L.)
*Eurasian Sparrowhawk, *Accipiter nisus* (L.)
Goshawk, *Accipiter gentilis* (L.)
Honey Buzzard, *Pernis apivorus* (L.) (1 specimen)
Hen Harrier, *Circus cyaneus* (L.) (1 specimen)

Falconidae, Falcons
  *Old World Kestrel, *Falco tinnunculus* L.
Phasianidae, Fowllike Birds and Pheasants
  *Domestic Fowl, *Gallus domesticus* L.
  Grey Partridge, *Perdix perdix* (L.)
  Common Quail, *Coturnix coturnix* (L.)
  Valley Quail, *Lophortyx californicus* (Shaw)
  *Chinese Painted Quail, *Excalfactoria chinensis* (L.)
  Himalayan Monal Pheasant, *Lophophorus impejanus* (Latham)
  Nepal Kalij, *Gennaeus leucomelanos* (Latham)
  Ring-necked Pheasant, *Phasianus colchicus* L.
  Golden Pheasant, *Chrysolophus pictus* (L.)
  *Reeve's Pheasant, *Syrmaticus reevesii* (J. E. Gray)
  Peacock-Pheasant, *Polyplectron spec.*
  Indian Peafowl, *Pavo cristatus* (L.)
Numididae, Guineafowl
  Helmeted Guineafowl, *Numida meleagris* L.
Gruidae, Cranes
  Demoiselle Crane, *Anthropoides virgo* (L.)
  Crowned Crane, *Balearica pavonina* (L.)
Rallidae, Rails
  Water Rail, *Rallus aquaticus* L.
  Common Moorhen, *Gallinula chloropus* (L.)
  *Coot, *Fulica atra* L.
  Allen's Gallinule, *Porphyrula alleni* (Thomson) (1 specimen)
Haematopodidae, Oystercatchers
  Oystercatcher, *Haematopus ostralegus* L.
Charadriidae, Plovers
  *Lapwing, *Vanellus vanellus* (L.)
  Golden Plover, *Pluvialis apricaria* (L.)
Scolopacidae, Woodcocks, Curlews and Sandpipers
  European Woodcock, *Scolopax rusticola* (L.)
  Common Curlew, *Numenius arquata* (L.)
  *Redshank, *Tringa totanus* (L.)
  Common Sandpiper, *Tringa hypoleucos* L.
Glareolidae, Pratincoles
  Egyptian Plover, *Pluvianus aegypticus* (L.) (1 specimen)
Laridae, Gulls
  Great Black-backed Gull, *Larus marinus* L.
  *Herring Gull, *Larus argentatus* Pontoppidan
  *Black-headed Gull, *Larus ridibundus* (L.)
Sternidae, Terns
  Common Tern, *Sterna hirundo* L.
  Roseate Tern, *Sterna dongallii* Montagu (1 specimen)
Alcidae, Auks
  *Razor-billed Auk, *Alca torda* L.
  *Common Murre, *Uria aalge* (Pontoppidan)
  Puffin, *Fratercula arctica* (L.)
Columbidae, Pigeons
  *Domestic Pigeon, *Columba domestica* L.
  Wood Pigeon, *Columba palumbus* L.
  Collared Turtle Dove, *Streptopelis decaocta* (Frivaldsky)
  Diamant Ground Dove, *Geopelia cuneata* (Latham)
Psittacidae, Parrots
  *Nymph Parrot, *Nymphicus hollandicus* (Kerr)
  Blue-fronted Parrot, *Amazona aestiva* (1 specimen)
  Lesser Lovebird, *Agapornis spec.*
  Western Rosella, *Platycercus icterotis* (Kuhl)

Red-backed Parrot, *Psephotus haematonotus* (Gould)
*Budgerigar, *Melopsittacus undulatus* (Shaw)
Cuculidae, Cuckoos
  Cuckoo, *Cuculus canorus* L.
Strigidae, Owls
  Barn Owl, *Tyto alba* (Scopoli)
  Little Owl, *Athene noctua* (Scopoli)
  Tawny Owl, *Strix aluco* L.
  Long-eared Owl, *Asio otus* (L.)
Apodidae, Swifts
  *Common Swift, *Apus apus* (L.)
Trochilidae, Hummingbirds
  *Ruby-topaz Hummingbird, *Chrysolampis mosquitus* (L.)
                        Agytria lactea
  *White-eared Hummingbird, *Hylocharis leucotis* (Vieillot)
  Black-white Hummingbird, *Melanotrochilus fuscus* (V.)
Alcedinidae, Kingfishers
  Kingfisher, *Alcedo atthis* (L.) (1 specimen)
Ramphastidae, Toucans
  Fisher Toucan, *Ramphastus sulfuratus* Lesson (1 specimen)
Picidae, Woodpeckers
  Great Spotted Woodpeckers, *Dendrocopos major* (L.)
Hirundinidae, Swallows
  Common Swallow, *Hirundo rustica* L.
Laniidae, Shrikes
  Red-backed Shrike, *Lanius collurio* L.
Bombycillidae, Waxwings
  Bohemian Waxwing, *Bombycilla garrulus* (L.)
Troglodytidae, Wrens
  Winter Wren, *Troglodytes troglodytes* (L.)
Muscicapidae, Flycatchers
  Savi's Warbler, *Locustella luscinioides* (Savi)
  *River Warbler, *Locustella fluviatilis* (Wolf)
  Blackcap, *Sylvia atricapilla* (L.)
  *Firecrest, *Regulus ignicapillus* (Temminck)
  Goldcrest, *Regulus regulus* (L.)
  *Redstart, *Phoenicurus phoenicurus* (L.)
  Robin, *Erithacus rubecula* (L.)
  Fieldfare, *Turdus pilaris* L.
  Song Trush, *Turdus philomelos* Brehm
  *Blackbird, *Turdus merula* L.
Paridae, Titmice
  Oxeye-tit, *Parus major* L.
Emberizidae, Buntings
  Yellowhammer, *Emberiza citrinella* L.
  Corn Bunting, *Emberiza calandra* L.
Fringillidae, Finches
  Cardinal, *Cardinalis cardinalis* (L.)
  *Greenfinch, *Carduelis chloris* (L.)
  *Goldfinch, *Carduelis carduelis* (L.)
  Redpoll, *Carduelis flammeus* (L.)
  Linnet, *Carduelis cannabina* (L.)
  Hawfinch, *Coccothraustes coccothraustes* (L.)
  Canary, *Serinus canaria* (L.)
Ploceidae, Weaverbirds
  *House Sparrow, *Passer domesticus* (L.)
  Orange Bishop, *Euplectes franciscanus* (Isert)
                Sitagra luteola (Lichtenstein)

Red-checked Cordon-bleu, *Granatina spec.*
Grey Waxbill, *Estrilda troglodytes* (Lichtenstein)
Crimson-rumped Waxbill, *Estrilda rhodopyga* Sundevall
Lavender Finch, *Estrilda caerulescens* (Vieillot)
Magpie Mannikin, *Spermestes fringilloides* (Lafresnaye)
Avadavat, *Amandava amandava* (L.)
African Silverbill, *Euodice cantans* (Gmelin)
Java Sparrow, *Padda oryzivora* (L.)
*Parrot Finch, *Erythrura spec.*
Paradise Widow, *Steganura paradisaea* (L.)
Zebra Finch, *Taeniopygia guttata* (Vieillot)
Sturnidae, Starlings
  *Starling, *Sturnus vulgaris* L.
  Long-tailed Glossy Starling, *Lamprotornis caudatus* (Müller)
Corvidae, Crows
  *Black-throated Jay, *Garrulus glandarius* (L.)
  Magpie, *Pica pica* (L.)
  Nutcracker, *Nucifraga caryocatactes* (L.)
  Jackdaw, *Corvus monedula* L.
  *Carrion Crow, *Corvus corone* L.

The systematic classification and the determination of these species—as far as it was not doubtlessly declared by the animal store—was practiced according to Gilliard and Steinbacher (1959), Alexander and Niethammer (1959), Scott and Klös (1961), Peterson, Mountfort, Hollom, and Niethammer (1965), Niethammer, Bauer, and Glutz von Blotzheim (1966, 1968, 1969) and Grzimek, Meise, Niethammer, Steinbacher, and Thenius (1968), Grzimek, Meise, Niethammer, and Steinbacher (1969, 1970).

The species listed above were injected and processed into lung-air sac casts, usually still connected to the skeleton. In the course of the intensive preparation the injection casts were then disconnected from the skeleton. Generally two or more specimens of each species were prepared. One specimen only was obtainable in a number of rare species; this is mentioned in the species list.

For the completion of the results obtained from the injection preparations the species marked by an asterisk were studied by intensive preparation. In the course of this preparation, the air sacs with their walls and the septa were systematically demonstrated, then especially the ostia of the bronchi into the air sacs. For these studies specimens were chosen that had died shortly before or could be obtained alive. These specimens were fixed with Bouin's solution and prepared in 80% ethanol. After demonstration of the air sacs, the lungs were taken out.

The walls of the air sacs and the septa were excised during the preparation, just as the wide membranous walls of the dorso- and ventrobronchi, and processed into membrane preparations. These membrane preparations were stained with chromotrop resorcin fuchsin according to Petry (1951), also partly with the trichrome stain according to Goldner and the azan stain according to Heidenhain (Romeis, 1948, §§ 1498, 1989), placed on a glass slide and covered with a coverslip.

Small pieces were taken from the removed lungs and small lungs were totally processed by the paraffin technique. The pieces were cut in such a manner, that all important structures, primary bronchus, dorso- and ventrobronchi, parabronchi and saccobronchi could be studied. The thickness of the sections varied between 5, 8 and 25 μ, at very important points series of sections were cut. The sections were stained with hematoxylin eosin, Goldner, azan and resorcin fuchsin nuclear fast red (Romeis, 1948, §§ 677, 1498, 1489, 1560).

In some species, mute swan, northern mallard, coot, domestic fowl, Reeve's pheasant, domestic pigeon, old world kestrel, black-headed gull, black-throated jay, house sparrow and blackbird, Berlin blue gelatine was injected into blood vessels.

In particular big species, mute swan, northern mallard and domestic fowl, the injections into the blood vessels were made in two colors, with solid red gelatine being injected into the pulmonary arteries; thus the topography of arteries and veins in the respiratory tissue mantle of the parabronchus could be studied. Frozen sections were made from pieces of these fixed and injected lungs. Single two colored vessel injections with technovit accompanied by simultaneous injection of the bronchial system with technovit in the mute swan and white stork were used to demonstrate the topography of the vessel tree in relation to the bronchial system.

In order to recognize the connections of the air capillaries, the lungs of the mute swan, northern mallard, domestic fowl, Reeve's pheasant, domestic pigeon, common buzzard, old world kestrel, black-headed gull, black-throated jay, carrion crow and blackbird after evacuation were covered with a very fine mixture of gelatine and Indian ink, which reached the last recesses of the air capillary network when the air pressure began to rise again. After fixation, frozen sections were made from pieces of these lungs. The method was however only successful when the pieces were frozen in fluid nitrogen.

The procurement of a part of the experimental material and the histological studies were carried out with a grant of Deutsche Forschungsgemeinschaft (Vogellunge — Du 50/1).

For the excellent drawings I am gratefully indebted to H. Hess of the Anatomical Institute Hamburg. Grateful acknowledgement are made to the Joachim Jungius-Gesellschaft der Wissenschaften Hamburg, which made possible the production of a portion of the drawings.

Notes on Terminology

The short, fixed terms that are used in the anatomical and physiological literature are maintained without any changes in the description of the different parts of the lung, the air sacs and the septa. This is valid for the designation of the bronchi too. The *"primary bronchus"* of current English authors (King, 1956; Salt and Zeuthen, 1960, and other authors) is termed mesobronchium in its whole length by Huxley (1882), accordingly mesobronchus by some other authors (Scheid and Piiper, 1970, and other authors). The primary bronchus is marked by a more or less distinct dilatation between the two branching groups of secondary bronchi, the vestibulum. In front of the vestibulum the *"ventrobronchi"* (Brandes, 1924) originate, the bronches diaphragmatiques of Sappey (1847), entobronchi (Gadow, 1891, and other authors) or mesiobronchi (Delphia, 1961). They are fixed by their names in the given position within the lung. The same is true for the *"dorsobronchi"* (Brandes, 1924) which are situated on the dorsolateral surface of the lung. Sappey (1847) named them bronches costales, Gadow (1891) and others ectobronchi. In both groups of these secondary bronchi the naming of the individual bronchi (Fischer, 1905) other than by number is omitted.

The *"laterobronchi"* (Locy and Larsell, 1916) could better be described by the term lateroventrobronchi (Delphia, 1961) but the shorter form is unequivocal considering the unambiguous terms of the two other groups of secondary bronchi. The tertiary bronchi of English speaking authors are similar to the smallest bronchial units which Huxley (1882) called *"parabronchi"*. This name is not only generally accepted but also of such typical character that it is by far superior to all such others as lung pipes of german authors (Scharnke, 1934), bronchial the naming of the individual bronchi (Fischer, 1905) other than by number is 1905).

The *"saccobronchi"* which were for the first described and named by Schulze (1910) have already been termed recurrent also by Schulze himself. They appeared as bronchi recurrentes in the literature (Juillet, 1912a, b) and, as a possibility to interpret the lung ventilation, they played a major part in the discussion of the lung function (Brandes, 1924; Dotterweich, 1930a, b; Vos, 1935). Since today that interpretation lacks any validity it is advantageous to return to the functionally neutral name saccobronchi (Scharnke, 1934; Salt and Zeuthen, 1960).

In naming the different air sacs the generally accepted topographical terms that symbolize the position in the trunk are maintained (Scharnke, 1934; Salt and Zeuthen, 1960). The *"cervical air sac"* corresponds to the reservoir cervical of Sappey (1847) and the saccus praebronchialis (Huxley, 1882). The impar *"interclavicular air sac"* is Sappey's (1847) reservoir interclaviculair and Huxley's (1882) saccus subbronchialis. The *"anterior thoracic air sac"* of Salt and Zeuthen (1960) is equivalent to Scharnke's (1934) prethoracic air sac, Huxley's (1882) saccus intermedius anterior and Sappey's (1847) reservoir diaphragmatique anterieur as well as to the saccus hepaticus anterior of other older authors. The terms for the *"posterior thoracic air sac"* are corresponding to the other names, consequently saccus intermedius posterior (Huxley, 1882) and reservoir diaphragmatique posterieur (Sappey, 1847). The *"abdominal air sac"* (Scharnke, 1934; Salt and Zeuthen, 1960) is called reservoir abdominal by Sappey (1847). Huxley, in his description of the air sacs of the kiwi as the last mentions the saccus posterior; basing on the comparative studies of this paper I am not sure whether Huxley has really seen an abdominal air sac in the kiwi (a matter that remains dubious in his description) and whether therefore his saccus posterior is homologous to the abdominal air sac of all other birds.

The openings or ostia into the individual air sacs are generally designated as the ostium of the corresponding air sac or as an opening into the corresponding air sac. An individual designation of the particular ostia of the primary, latero-, ventro- and saccobronchi without direct relation to the corresponding air sac only leads to great confusion as is demonstrated by the work of Fischer (1905).

Corresponding to the membranes that divide the abdominal cavity of birds the term diaphragm is preferably used: pulmonary diaphragm and abdominal diaphragm of Salt and Zeuthen (1960) or horizontal and oblique diaphragm in the German literature (Gadow, 1891, and other authors). The horizontal diaphragm also called transverse or pulmonal diaphragm (Gadow, 1891) is Sappey's diaphragme pulmonaire (1847) and the diaphragmite antérieur of Milne-Edwards (1865) and the diaframma ornitico of Bertelli (1898, 1905). Huxley (1882) and Butler (1889) called the pulmonal diaphragm pulmonary aponeurosis, Beddard (1896) horizontal septum. This *"horizontal septum"* is demonstrated to be the dorsal part of the postpulmonary septum, by embryological and comparative studies of Poole (1909). The ventral portion of the postpulmonary septum is the oblique diaphragm, the diaphragme thoraco-abdominale of Sappey (1847) which is called the *"oblique septum"* by Huxley (1882), Butler (1889) and Beddard (1896). Since the mammalian diaphragm is a special structure in relation to its position and development and since it definitely is not completely homologous to the membranes of the avian body and also since functional relations cannot be demonstrated between these two structures I am inclined to join Huxley (1882), Butler (1889) and Beddard (1896) in speaking of the horizontal as well as of the oblique septum. By this nomenclature the two septa are also related to the varying septa that divide the abdominal cavity of varans and crocodiles, and that are the phylogenetical precursors of the postpulmonary septum of birds. The postpulmonary septum then gives rise to the horizontal and oblique septum.

2*

Huxley (1882) gives the cavities of the avian body which arise between the septa, names of their own. He divides the whole thoracoabdominal cavity into a *"cavum respiratorium"* in front of and dorsal to the oblique septum and a *"cavum cardioabdominale"* which, behind and ventral to the oblique septum, contains the bulk of intestines including the heart. The cavum respiratorium is divided by the horizontal septum into the dorsally situated *"cavum pulmonale"*, and the *"cavum subpulmonale"* lying underneath, which, with the exception of the abdominal air sacs, contains all the other air sacs. The abdominal air sacs are lying in the cavum cardioabdominale — a fact that was unknown to Huxley who described the kiwi air sacs (1882). The use of Huxley's terms renders possible a very short and precise description of topographical relations.

Results

Structure of the Thoracoabdominal Wall

For a complete comprehension of the position of the lungs and air sacs in the body as well as functional aspects it becomes necessary to give an introduction into the anatomy of the trunk wall. Besides material of the author, the works of Fürbringer (1888, 1902), Gadow (1891), Remane (1936), Bellairs and Jenkin (1960), Berger (1960) and George and Berger (1966) mostly however the excellent study of Zimmer (1935) form the basis of this introduction.

The thoracic region of the trunk is formed in most families of birds by 3–10, mostly however by 5 or 6 vertebrae. The thoracic vertebrae are connected to the sternum by their ribs which are subdivided into a dorsal curved vertebral rib and an adjoining straight sternal rib (Figs. 1–3, 5–8). The last or the two last cervical vertebrae also regularly bear vertebral ribs, which have no adjoining sternal ribs and thus no connection to the sternum. Besides, the anterior 1–3, sometimes four vertebrae of the synsacrum, which directly follow the rib bearing thoracic vertebrae, usually display fully developed ribs. They too are consistent of a vertebral and a sternal rib and are connected to the sternum (Figs. 1–3, 5, 7, 8); only the last of these ribs may show a free ending as a vertebral rib or may, with its sternal rib, connect to the preceding sternal rib (Figs. 5a, c, 6a, b).

The abdominal region, adjoining to the thoracic, is formed dorsally by the pelvis, a fusion of ilium, ischium and pubic bone with the synsacrum, which consists of the lumbal, sacral and the first caudal vertebrae. Mostly, the last thoracic vertebrae are also incorporated into this fusion. The pelvis has the configuration of a long saddlelike roof, the ridge of which is formed by the vertebrae and the sides by the pelvic bones. At about the middle of the ilium the anterior ends of the ischium and pubis fuse with the ilial bone thus forming the acetabular fossa for the head of the femur. In diving birds the pelvis is extremely narrow arising from their leg position and body posture (Fig. 1), while in most species it is wider, especially behind the hip joint. There, ischium and pubis often arch across the whole dorsal abdomen (Figs. 2, 6a–c). The cranial portion of the free coccygeal vertebral column covers the most caudal part of the abdominal cavity. Pubis and ischium surround the cloaca in a very different manner in different species, or end in the lateral abdominal wall, never forming a symphysis. The remaining parts of the lateral and ventral abdominal wall contain no skeletal elements (Figs. 2, 5a–c, 6a–c, 8).

The predominantly swimming, partly also diving birds, penguins and loons, auks and ducks, have a longer, stretched body. Their trunk wall structure is characterized by a larger number of ribs and their vertebral ribs pass from the thoracic vertebrae obliquely into a ventrocaudal direction. They join the sternal ribs in an acute angle, at a line about the border between the middle and lower third of the lateral trunk wall, between the transverse processes of the vertebral column and the lateral margin of the sternum. The sternal ribs pass obliquely in a ventrocranial direction, forming joints with the lateral margin of the sternum. Thus a larger part of the lateral abdominal wall is supported by ribs. At the same time, the wide sternum is very long and reaches very far caudally in these species, so that a large part of the ventral abdominal wall possesses skeletal elements. The sternal ribs articulate along the greater part of the sternal sides. The long sternum lies mostly parallel to the vertebral column or forms only a very acute angle with it (Figs. 1, 5a–c, 7a, b, 8).

Contrary to the swimming birds, the terrestrial birds that are the majority and which either run or fly — as does the greater number — display a broad, but relatively short sternum, which forms a wider angle with the vertebral column. In these species the ribs have been developed as far as the anterior end of the ilium only; the vertebral ribs pass almost perpendicular to the vertebral column in a lateroventral direction and, in an obtuse angle, form joints with the sternal ribs. In these species too the joints between vertebral and sternal ribs lie at a level between the middle and lower third of the lateral thoracic wall, this line forming an acute angle with both the vertebral column and the sternal margin. Mostly the joints of the sternal ribs are crowded together at the cranial margin of the sternum. It follows that the lateral and ventral portions of the abdomen of terrestrial birds is free of skeletal parts (Figs. 2, 6a–c).

The thoracic vertebrae are characterized by vertebral bodies which are relatively high and often so narrow that the articular surfaces markedly project to the sides. The parapophyses, which joint with the capitula of the ribs, have risen to the basis of the neural arches. The diapophyses are generally well developed as processus transversi and shifted towards the basis of the spinal thorns, so that they often form a sharp right angle with the processus spinosi. Then they are situated in the same plane as the almost horizontally formed pre- and postzygapophyses. The ribs normally have tubercula of such marked prominence that these are provided with a longer neck, and one is inclined to speak of bicipital ribs. The articular surfaces for these tubercula lie at the peak of the processus transversi. It follows that the axis for motions of the vertebral ribs is fixed; it passes through both articular surfaces and forms an angle with the axis of the vertebral column that is about 90 degrees for the most cranial and a little less than 90° for the following ribs (measured caudally between ribs and vertebral column). The angle size decreases from rib to rib in a caudal direction (Fig. 7a, b).

The axes of the joints between sternal ribs and sternal margin are formed in a very similar way. Thus the point at which vertebral articulates with the sternal rib may move ventrally and a little laterally, while the ribs in the dorsal

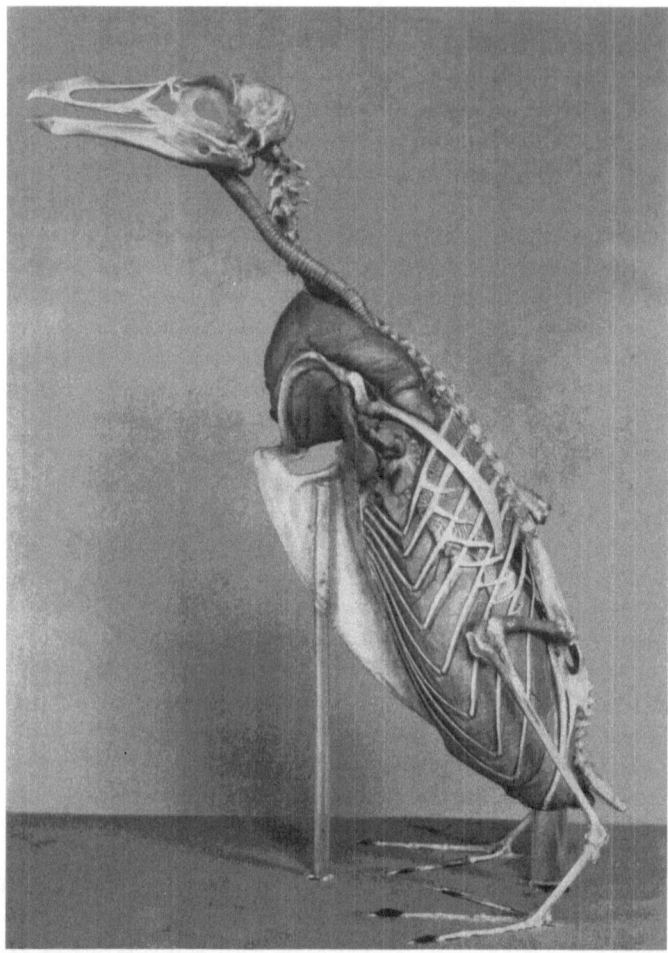

Fig. 1. Skeleton lung air sac preparation of a razor-billed auk, *Alca torda*, seen from lateral. *Type of the swimming form.* Sternum reaching far caudally. Vertebral and sternal ribs articulate forming an acute angle with each other. Interclavicular air sac overlaps the clavicle far towards ventral. Scapula lies on the vertebral ribs with long uncinate processes. Wings have been disarticulated in the shoulder joint. ×0.4

thoracic region shift themselves practically only parallel in a cranial direction. With the rotation of the articular axis of the ribs towards the pelvis, the outward motion of the ribs, at constant forward motion, increases so much the more, the more caudally they are situated. Through the position of the angle between vertebral and sternal rib the sternum is displaced from the vertebral column, cranially a little only, caudally in increasing amounts, so that the angle between sternum and vertebral column increases. This is equally true for the terrestrial as well as for the swimming form of the body of birds (Figs. 1–3, 5a–c, 6a–c, 7a, b, 8).

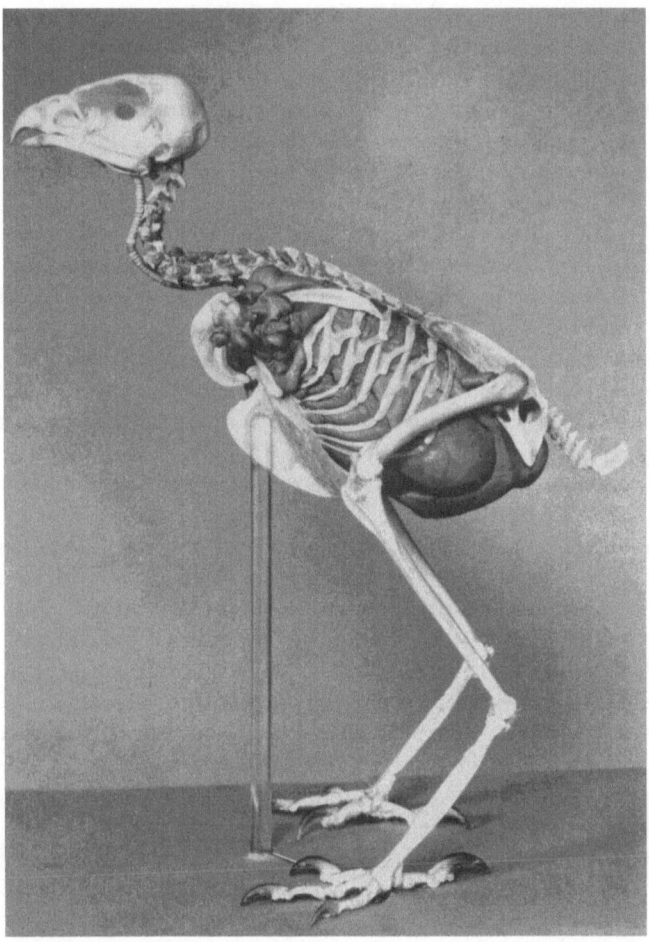

Fig. 2. Skeleton lung air sac preparation of a common buzzard, *Buteo buteo*, seen from lateral. *Type of the flying form.* Short sternum which forms a greater angle with the vertebral column. Vertebral and sternal ribs articulate in the form of an obtuse angle. Well developed clavicle overlaps the interclavicular air sac with its axillary diverticula which surround the coracoid and anterior sacpula, too. Scapula lies on the vertebral ribs with small but solid processus uncinati. Wings have been disarticulated in the shoulder joint. ×0.4

The thoracic vertebrae are very little mobile against each other. The mobility may be completely lost in the middle 3 or 4 thoracic vertebrae, when these have grown together into a notarium or os dorsale, which can be found in some families. The thoracic vertebrae often on their ventral side bear high but very narrow processes, the hypapophyses, which reach their greatest height in the middle of the thoracic vertebral column and become lower in both cranial and caudal direction. Mostly, they are connected by a membrane into a median wall, more seldom by a bony plate, which subdivides the dorsal thoracic cavity at the midline (Fig. 7a, b). The thoracic cavity then encloses the narrow bodies

of the thoracic vertebrae on both sides and, including the region of the neural
arches in its total length, directly reaches beneath the processus transversi.

The ribs lying flatly within the thoracic wall give off the stalked tubercula
in a dorsal direction for an articulation with the processus transversi and, beginning at this splitting, cut deep into the free dorsal thoracic cavity. These
craniocaudally flattened ribs reach with their capitulum the parapophyses at
the side of the vertebral body. The thorax in its dorsal part is formed in such
a manner by these ribs, arcuately reaching the vertebral bodies, that it cannot
be compressed in a transverse direction (Fig. 7 a, b). This has the effect that
in all birds, especially prominent in good flyers, the dorsal thoracic cavity is
subdivided by the ribs into individual compartments.

This construction of the dorsal thorax also extends to the last, rib bearing
cervical vertebrae and to the caudal, rib bearing thoracic vertebrae that are
incorporated into the pelvic formation. The last ribs, originating beneath the
ilium are generally not articulated but completely grown together. They are
so thin and elastic that they can follow the motions of the abdominal wall without
difficulties. This elaboration of the dorsal thoracic cavity is found in all birds,
independent of the type of function to which they belong. Differences can be
found only in the form of the hypapophyses, which can be of variable height
and which also lack completely in a number of species.

The ribs are connected to each other by the external and internal intercostal
muscles. The latter bring the ribs close to the vertebral column, reduce the angle
between vertebral and sternal ribs and move the sternum in a dorsal direction.
By this fixed possibility of rib mobility the dorsoventral and transverse diameter of the trunk and its total volume are reduced. Exactly antagonistic is
the work of the Mm. intercostales externi which partly insert at the processus
uncinati of the vertebral ribs – so very characteristic of birds – as Mm. appendicocostales (Fig. 3 b). By this effective mode of insertion they have received a very
favourable lever arm and are therefore able to practise a movement much stronger
than a corresponding amount of Mm. intercostales externi. These muscles reach
their highest development in species with long processus uncinati as socalled
Mm. interappendiculares, if they insert from the following on the foregoing
processus uncinati. This high development of the processes is characteristic of
the swimming form (Zimmer, 1935). An effective dilatation of the thorax is
possible by the action of the Mm. intercostales externi and especially of the
Mm. appendicocostales, and, if present, the Mm. interappendiculares (Fig. 3 b).
This dilatation extends into the abdomen in relation to the caudal extension of
the ribs, which means that it is especially marked in swimming forms. The
trunk dilatation is aided by the Mm. levatores costarum, costocoracoideus and
costosternales (Fig. 3 b), as well as by the Mm. scalenus and teres. More muscles
with dilating function on the thorax are not existent, mainly the so-called auxiliary
respiratory muscles are lacking.

The whole abdominal wall, as far as it is not carried by the ribs, is formed
by the Mm. transversus abdominis, obliquus abdominis internus and obliquus
abdominis externus, quadratus lumborum, iliocostalis, rectus abdominis and
transversus analis. They originate from the sternum, the ribs and the pelvis.
Whichever portions of them step into action, singular or combined, they always

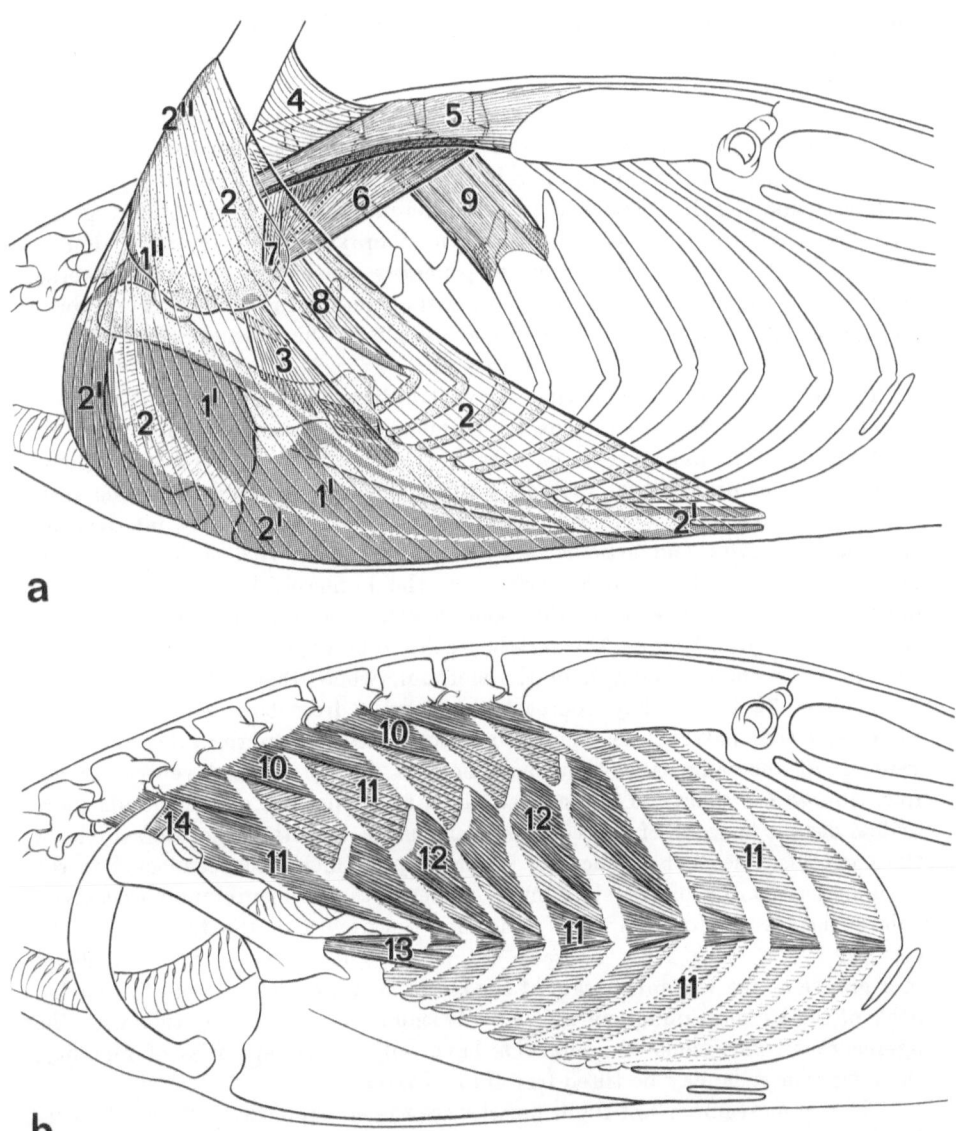

Fig. 3a and b. Mute swan, *Cygnus olor*, locomotor system of the shoulder and the thorax. a) Areas of origin and insertion of the shoulder girdle muscles are dotted. *1'* area of origin of the M. supracoracoideus on the sternum, coracoid and membrana coracoclavicularis, *1''* insertion at the humerus, *2* M. pectoralis pars thoracicus with *2'* its area of origin on the clavicle, membrana coracoclavicularis and sternum and *2''* insertion at the deltoid crest of the humerus. The M. pectoralis p. thoracicus passes freely mobil across the ventral ribs, separated by loose connective tissue. *3* M. coracobrachialis posterior with area of origin and insertion covering the M. sternocoracoideus. *4* M. latissimus dorsi pars anterior, *5* M. latissimus dorsi pars posterior, *6* M. dorsalis scapulae, *7* M. serratus profundus, *8* M. serratus anterior, *9* M. serratus posterior. b) Inspiratory muscles of the thorax. *10* Mm. levatores costarum, *11* Mm. intercostales externi as well as the *12* Mm. appendicocostales originating from the former, *13* Mm. costocoracoideus and costosternalis, *14* M. scalenus only are able to reduce the abdominal volume. Therefore they can only aid the Mm. intercostales interni and by this they represent the group of compressors of the thoracoabdominal cavity.

The musculature that moves the femur against the pelvis, originates exclusively from the rigid pelvis. Thus their function has no influence on the trunk movements. The position of the legs limits only the widening of the trunk.

The shoulder girdle is constructed in a different manner. The sternum together with the ribs forms the ventral wall of the thorax and the ventral abdomen. The cranial thoracic aperture is formed primarily by the last cervical vertebrae, the vertebral ribs originating from them and the inferior part of the first vertebral-sternal rib pair together with the cranial margin of the sternum. This primary cranial thoracic aperture is always very wide.

The sternum is at the same time the ventral impar part of the shoulder girdle which is composed of the coracoids, the scapulae and the clavicles joined together to the furcula. The flat, narrow, long scapula lies parallel to the vertebral column on the anterior dorsolateral thoracic wall, in an oblique plane extending from dorsomedial to ventrolateral. The anterior end of the scapula by far overlaps the thoracic cavity and articulates with the coracoid. With their articulating portion both form the glenoid surface for the humerus. Both wide and well developed coracoids pass from this point which is situated far in front of the first rib and a little beneath the vertebral column plane, in a ventrocaudal direction into the anterior margin of the sternum, where they articulate (Figs. 1, 3a, b, 5a–c, 7a, b, 8). They approach the sternum from both sides in a V-like figure and thus narrow the cranial thoracic aperture from the sides and from ventral. At the same time they incorporate a cavity situated ventral to the first rib into the thorax. The clavicles which form the fork of the furcula more or less distant in front of the coracoids, articulate with the craniodorsal end of the coracoids. The peak of the fork is normally ligamentously connected to the variably long carina of the sternum. Together with the membrana coracoclavicularis the furcula forms another balconied outgrowth of the thorax into the cervical region (Figs. 1–3a, b, 5a–c, 7a, b, 8). The coracoids are articulated in a groove at the ventral margin of the sternum, which passes from the medial peak of the sternum obliquely into a ventrocaudal direction. Together with the ligamentous connections the coracoids have only small capacities of mobility, their superior ends may be tilted forward and lateral.

The two most important flight muscles are the M. supracoracoideus ("M. pectoralis minor") and the M. pectoralis pars thoracicus ("M. pectoralis maior"). The M. supracoracoideus originates (differently in different species) from the dorsal portion of the carina sterni, from the medial part of the corpus sterni, adjoining to the carina, from the inferior part of the coracoid and from the membrana coracoclavicularis, partly also from the inferior clavicle (Fig. 3a). Its tendon inserts, after passage through the canalis triosseus craniomedial to the shoulder joint, dorsally at the anterior end of the head of the humerus. Therefore the M. supracoracoideus is the strong winglifter. The wing is pulled down by the M. pectoralis pars thoracicus, which totally overlaps the M. supracoracoideus and originates from the parts of the sternum remaining uncovered, and its carina, the coracoid, the clavicle and the membrana coracoclavicularis

(Fig. 3a). According to its function as the main flight muscle, the M. pectoralis is the largest and strongest muscle of the avian body in all birds capable of flying. The enormous development of the Mm. supracoracoideus and pectoralis p. thoracicus must be regarded as the cause for the widening of the sternum and the development of its carina for the enlargement of the area of muscle origin.

It is characteristic for the development of these two flight muscles that their area of origin has never been extended over the margins of the sternum on to the ribs; rather the sternum is developed in length and width according to the area of origin. This becomes especially clear in highly specialized groups as the fowllike birds, which have a sternum that, besides its numerous large caudal incisures or foramina has a lateral processus obliquus (Stresemann, 1927–1934; Remane, 1936; George and Berger, 1966) that is situated far dorsally above the ribs (Fig. 6a). The ribs are separated by loose connective tissue from this process and can move independently. The parts of the M. pectoralis p. thoracicus originating from this process pass over the ventral thorax on their way to the humerus. In this region, too, loose connective tissue can readily be found, even then, when the lateral processes of the sternum are lacking and the M. pectoralis, originating from the sternal margin only, passes to the humerus across the ventral ribs (Fig. 3a). Between the lateral part of the M. pectoralis and the ribs lies not only connective tissue but also the M. obliquus abdominis externus, which inserts at the lateral sternal margin and belongs to the locomotor system of the thoracoabdominal cavity. The loose connective tissue isolates the movements of the M. pectoralis against those of the rib cage. This is substantially aided by the development of the large coracoid directly in the direction of pulling function of the M. pectoralis towards the shoulder joint (Fig. 3a) and by the fact that the pull of the M. pectoralis is widely cushioned by the sternum, the origin of the muscle.

During the action of the M. pectoralis p. thoracicus, during the stroke down of the wing, the coracoid experiences a slight forward and outward motion, corresponding to its small mobility, which is reversed during the lift off of the wing by contraction of the M. supracoracoideus (Zimmer, 1935). These movements do not influence the rib cage. The clavicles, that are well developed as the furcula, together with the membrana coracoclavicularis serve as enlargement of the anterior area of origin for both flight muscles. On one hand the scapula is the origin of the muscles that regulate the movements of the humerus, as the Mm. dorsalis scapulae and subscapularis (Fig. 3a).

On the other hand the muscles originating from the scapula serve as connection between thorax and shoulder girdle. These small muscles in part pass to the vertebral column as Mm. rhomboidei superficiales and essentially seem to fix the scapula at the vertebral column. The second group of these muscles is composed of the Mm. serratus superficialis pars posterior and pars anterior and serratus profundus. They originate laterally at the anterior or posterior ribs beneath the processus uncinati (Fig. 3a). The different parts of the M. latissimus dorsi and the pars metapatagialis of the M. serratus superficialis have hardly any effects on the movements of the thorax because of their very weak development.

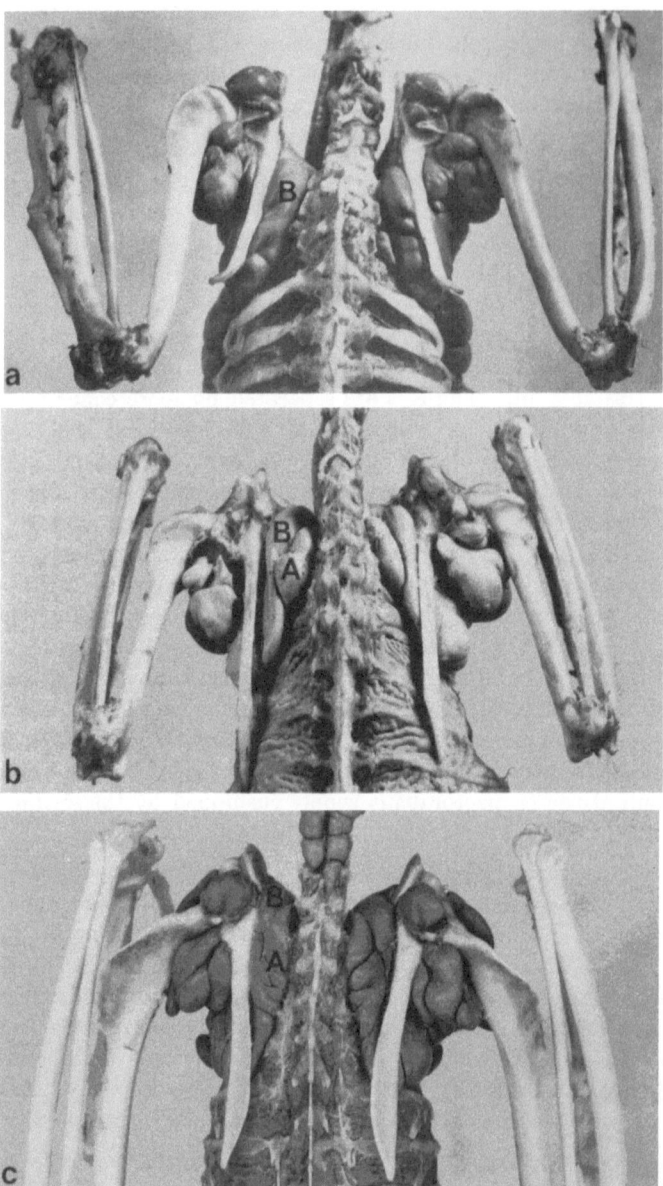

Fig. 4a–c. Shoulder regions of skeleton lung air sac preparations seen from dorsal. The anterior portion of the shoulder girdle is isolated from the anterior thorax by diverticula of the cervical and interclavicular air sacs. Around the shoulder joint lie the axillary diverticula of the interclavicular air sac. Beneath the ribs the bronchi of the lungs are seen. a) Great spotted woodpecker, *Dendrocopos major*, ×1.4. Only diverticula of the interclavicular air sac (*B*) lie between shoulder girdle and thorax. b) Starling, *Sturnus vulgaris*, ×1.3. A smaller diverticulum of the cervical (*A*) and a larger of the interclavicular air sac (*B*) are exhibited between shoulder girdle and thorax. c) Goshawk, *Accipiter gentilis*, ×0.7. A large diverticulum of the cervical (*A*) and a small of the interclavicular air sac (*B*) are seen between shoulder girdle and thorax

Considering the articulations and the muscular connections between thorax and shoulder girdle, it can be seen that during movements of the thorax, the sternum with the shoulder girdle is tilted against the vertebral column, the point of rotation of this angular motion being situated in the region of the shoulder joint (Fig. 8). This point of rotation is formed not only by the rib movements but also by the muscular fixation of the scapula. The scapula musculature in part belongs to that group which moves the thorax.

As already explained: the motions of the pelvic extremity do not at all influence the motions of the trunk wall. The movements of the wings also, by the arrangement of skeletal elements and muscles have no influence on the motions of the thoracic wall. The movements of the shoulder joints in a lateral direction during the wing motion, as observed by Zimmer (1935), does also have no influence on the thoracic wall, as Zimmer still believed possible, for a well developed diverticulum of the cervical and/or interclavicular air sac can be found between the dorsal part of the coracoid and the anterior scapula on one side and the anterior cranial thoracic wall on the other side in all well flying species. This diverticulum divides these two structures and allows them unimpaired mobility (Figs. 1, 2, 4–6).

The highly differentiated locomotor system of birds displays three primarily independent locomotion apparatuses in the region of the trunk: one for the wings (Fig. 3a); one for the legs and one for the thoracoabdominal cavity (Fig. 3b). The expansion of the abdominal cavity is caused by the angular motion of the sternum against the vertebral column — as described above — through a point of rotation near the shoulder joint and by the outward motion of the ribs (Fig. 8). The expansion gradually increases, starting at the plane of the shoulder joint where it is equal to zero, in a caudal direction, to reach its greatest extent at the end of the rib carrying abdominal wall and at the caudal end of the sternum or even farther caudally (Fig. 8). The punctum fixum of the trunk is of importance for a discussion of these trunk actions, which — as will be seen later — serve as inspiratory and retrograde expiratory motions. In the standing position the trunk hangs on the pelvis and the thoracic vertebral column rigidly affixed to it. Then the sternum moves against this fixed axis, the gravity, acting on the freely mobile content of the abdominal cavity, aiding the inspiratory movement. If the bird is sitting on the carina sterni, if it swims or hangs on the wings during flight and therefore in the shoulder girdle, the trunk always lies on the sternum and during inspiratory motions the vertebral column with the pelvis must be lifted against gravity.

Position and Form of the Lungs

The lungs of birds are symmetrically structured and they occupy the dorsal part of the thoracic cavity. The lungs are compactly and uniformly constructed and cannot be subdivided macroscopically, they are not divided into lobes. They regularly reach the first cranial rib which is only developed as a vertebral rib. Caudally the lungs generally extend as far as the cranial margin of the ilium, or just beneath it (Figs. 1, 2, 5a–c, 6a–c). Consequently they do not extend as far as the last rib which lies farther caudally under the ilium. In individual species the lungs reach farther caudally, almost as far as the level of the hip

joint: in storks, geese and hoatzins. In the storks the lungs even overlap the
last rib. Cranially the lungs in these species, too, reach the first rib, which is
therefore a character common to all birds. The lungs of the species mentioned
last are, in spite of their extension far into the pelvis, not longer than those
of other species, the storks even have especially short and thickset lungs. This
indicates that beyond the rough classification of types of body forms in a terrestrial and a swimming form, a surprising deviation of these types regarding the
proportional arrangement of the individual structure elements exists (Figs. 5a–c,
6a–c), the correlation of which to the specially developed environmental and
functional types of the particular species is still unknown.

The lungs lie close to the dorsolateral thoracic wall so that they enclose
those parts of the ribs which pass through the dorsal thoracic cavity to the
vertebral bodies (Fig. 7a, b). In that way the dorsomedial lung margins are
subdivided into regular sections by the rib incisures (Figs. 19a, 20b, 21a, 22a, b).
Medially the lungs annex directly to the vertebral bodies and the often existent
medial septum which is formed by the hypapophyses (Fig. 7a, b). Touching the
inferior margin of this septum the lungs usually conclude their dorsoventral
extension. In a number of species the lungs overlap even this bony inferior
margin in varying degrees; then a membranous septum is found between the
two lungs. The lungs display their greatest dorsoventral extension at the border
of the anterior and middle third or also a little closer to the midline (Figs. 19b,
20b, 21b, 22b). From this point of their greatest thickness the lungs continually
become thinner, and lower in both cranial and caudal direction. Corresponding
to the thickness of the lung at its medial margin which at first increases and
then decreases in a craniocaudal direction, passes the inferior margin of the vertebral bodies or the septum that is formed by the hypapophyses (Fig. 7a, b).
The hypapophyses, partly very marked, reach their greatest height at the border
between the anterior and middle third of the lung and very rapidly decrease
in height in both cranial and caudal direction.

At the lateral thoracic wall the lung with its ventral margin reaches a little
farther down in a ventral direction than with its medial margin. This is the
reason why the inferior surface of the lung slopes from medial to lateral a little
outward and ventral. The deepest point is situated at the lateral margin about
at the middle of the lung, normally just above the joints between 2nd and 3rd
vertebral and sternal rib. From there the ventral margin of the lung rises steeply
in a cranial direction, to go almost straight to the anterior lung peak that lies
directly beside the vertebral column. The ventral margin of the lung passes,
steadily ascending, in a caudal direction as far as laterally beneath the anterior
ilium (Figs. 5a–c, 6a–c). Caudally the lung is limited by a line running exactly
perpendicular towards the vertebral column. Through this margin the lung
receives an almost triangular shape, the caudal peak lacking (Figs. 19a, b, 20a, c,
21a, c, 22a, c, 28a, b, 29a–c). One side of the triangle lies close to the vertebral
column. Opposite at the thoracic wall, the deepest point of the lung is localized,
which at the same time is corresponding to the greatest extension of thickness.
Thus the line of greatest thickness on the inferior surface of the lung runs from
medial starting at the border between anterior and middle third, to the middle
of the lateral margin, consequently into a caudolateral and ventral direction.

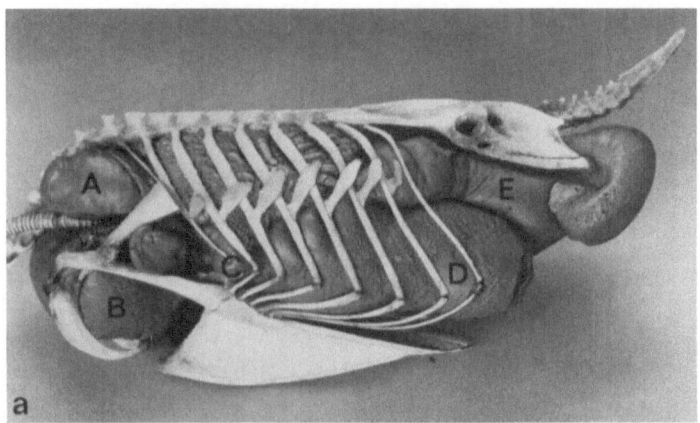

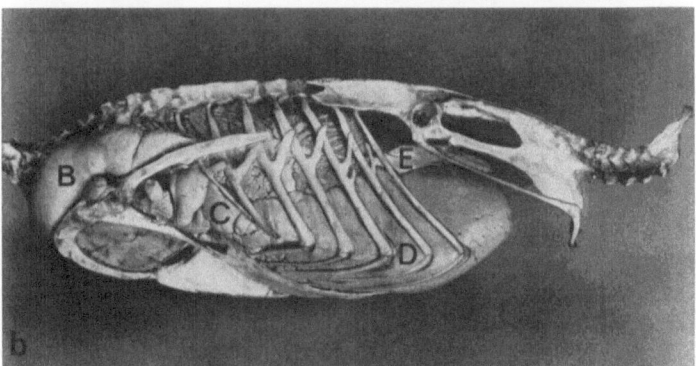

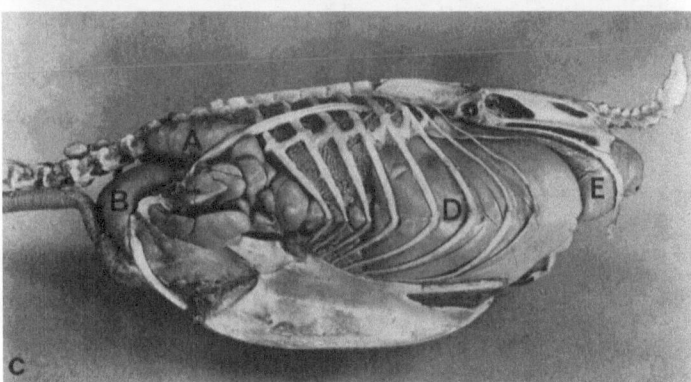

Fig. 5a–c. Skeleton lung air sac preparation seen from lateral, left side. Various swimming forms. Vertebral and sternal ribs articulate in an acute angle. Sternum reaching far caudally, the posterior thoracic air sac is always very large (*D*). The clavicula is always overlapped by the interclavicular air sac. a) Rockhopper penguin, *Eudyptes cristatus*, ×0.4. The broad scapula is cut off, broad uncinate processes. b) Green cormorant, *Phalacrocorax aristotelis*, ×0.4. The cervical air sac is covered by the interclavicular sac (*B*). c) Tufted duck, *Aythya fuligula*, ×0.5. Large axillary diverticula (*B*) around the shoulder joint. *A* cervical, *B* interclavicular, *C* anterior, and *D* posterior thoracic, *E* abdominal air sac

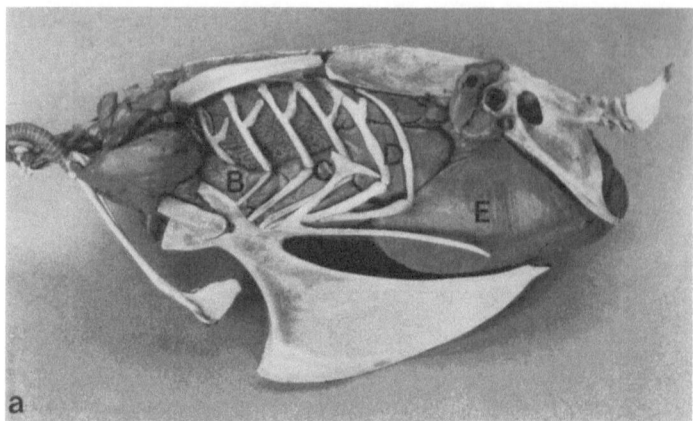

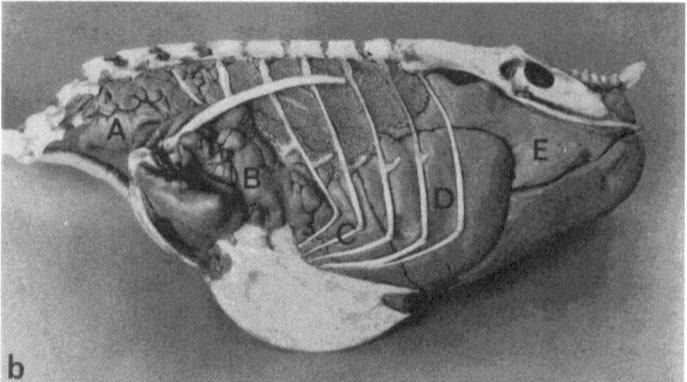

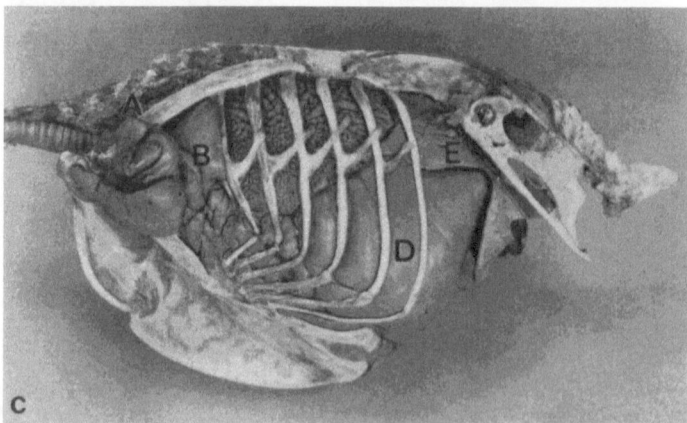

Fig. 6a–c. Skeleton lung air sac preparation seem from lateral, left side. Various terrestrial and flying forms. Vertebral and sternal ribs articulate in a right or obtuse angle. Well developed axillary diverticula of the interclavicular air sac (*B*) around the shoulder joint. The posterior thoracic air sac is of very different size. The proportions of the trunk markedly differ. a) Ring-necked pheasant, *Phasianus colchicus*, ×0.5. Very small posterior thoracic air sac (*D*). b) Grey heron, *Ardea cinerea*, ×0.4. Larger posterior thoracic air sac (*D*). c) Carrion crow, *Corvus corone*, ×0.7. Very large posterior thoracic air sac (*D*). *A* cervical, *C* anterior thoracic, *E* abdominal air sac

In the middle of this inferior surface line of greatest thickness of the lung lies the lung hilus (Figs. 19b, 20b, c, 21b, c, 22b, c, 28a, b, 29a–c).

A cross section through the lung at any level has a cuneate shape, the basis of which lies at the medial septum of the thorax (vertebral bodies and hypapophyses) and the peak of which lies close to the lateral thoracic wall which has the ventrally curved cuneate surface annexed to it (Figs. 16a–h, 17a–h). This form is characteristic for all avian lungs, the individual species differ only in the proportional arrangement. The penguin lungs are more stretched, longer yet not so wide and also not so thick (Figs. 20a–c, 28a); in contrast, the lungs of storks and herons are especially short yet very high (Fig. 21a–c), while the lungs of grebes show a special development in width, at the same time having a moderate extension in length and thickness. Essentially, the different species contrast only in the different proportions of the thorax. Only the extension of the laterocaudal part of the lung is determined by its internal structure, as can be shown by the differences in the individual species (Figs. 20a, 21a, 22a, 23a–c, 25a–c).

The ostia of the bronchial tree of the avian lung into the large air sacs lie in the inferior surface of the lung. For once they exist as openings into the interclavicular and anterior thoracic air sac directly medial to the hilus of the lung (Figs. 19b, 20c, 21c, 22c, 28a, b, 29a–c). Variably distant from the cranial lung tip, near the medial inferior margin lies the ostium into the cervical air sac. The great ostium into the posterior thoracic air sac is situated at the posterior lateral margin of the inferior lung surface (Figs. 19b, 20c, 21c, 22c, 28a, b, 29a–c). In the short, caudal margin of the lung, generally situated laterally, the ostium into the abdominal air sac is found. These ostia occupy the same positions in all birds, differences are only due to proportional shifts of the total form of the lung (Figs. 19–22, 28, 29). In species of higher systematical position the ostia into the posterior thoracic and into the abdominal air sac are oblique funnel shaped dilatations. In song birds the ostium into the posterior thoracic air sac is divided into two openings, one situated lateral at the lung margin and one medial, situated about at the middle of the posterior inferior lung surface (Figs. 22c 29c). In all species an additional ostium of varying size for the anterior thoracic and for the interclavicular air sac, which is situated at the anterior lateral lung margin, is added to these air sac ostia (Figs. 21c, 22c, 28b, 29a–c).

Organization of the Thoracoabdominal Cavity

The thoracoabdominal cavity of birds is on both sides subdivided in a number of completely separated chambers by the horizontal and oblique septum. This subdivision must be understood to originate from the changing septations of the body cavity in various lizards, especially varans, and mostly in crocodiles. Homologies of these septa to the mammalian diaphragm cannot be established. It has not been investigated as yet whether homologies exist between portions of the diaphragm, which are of totally different origin ontogenetically, and portions of the horizontal and oblique septum. The diaphragm of mammals is a special development which originates from other groups of reptiles. This is the reason why I will avoid the term diaphragm for these septa.

There is no simple division of the visceral cavity in a thoracic and an abdominal cavity in birds. The terms thoracic and abdominal cavity, used in the literature and in the further description are therefore sometimes ambiguous. Thoracic cavity is the cavity of the thoracic trunk region, between the caudal cervical and the thoracic vertebral column and the sternum. The abdominal cavity is the remaining posterior cavity of the trunk, which is covered dorsally by the pelvis but, laterally, may often carry ribs very far caudally and likewise, ventrally the caudal part of a very long sternum (Figs. 1, 5a–c).

Besides this regional use of the terms thoracic and abdominal, they are also used according to their essential contents. So, the room ventral and caudal to the oblique septa, containing liver, gizzard, intestinal tract, and urogenital system is the abdominal cavity. For practical purposes it is subdivided into an anterior, containing liver and gizzard, just above the sternum, and a posterior abdominal cavity, containing intestines, urogenital system and abdominal air sacs. The thoracic cavity remains as a room for the lung and the rest of the great air sacs, and therefore is situated not only cranial but in part also dorsal and lateral to the abdominal cavity (Figs. 16a–h, 17a–h).

This division of the visceral cavity in relation to its content corresponds to the classification and designation by Huxley (1882). He describes the space in front of and dorsal to the oblique septa as the cavum respiratorium, which often projects far into the abdominal cavity (Figs. 7a, b, 11, 13, 14, 15, 16a–h, 17a–h). The cavum cardioabdominale of Huxley begins like a pointed bag already at the anterior end of the sternum and expands until it occupies the whole visceral cavity in the region of the posterior abdomen (Figs. 7a, b, 11, 12, 14, 16a–h, 17a–h). It contains all viscera including the heart and the abdominal air sacs (Figs. 9, 10a, 11, 12–15, 16a–h, 17a–h). The cavum respiratorium contains the rest of the air sacs and the lungs which lie in its dorsal part and are separated from the air sacs by the horizontal septum (Figs. 7a, b, 11, 13, 15, 16a–h, 17a–h).

I. The Horizontal Septum of the Lung

The total inferior surface of the lung is directly covered by the horizontal septum, a well developed aponeurosis. This horizontal septum originates from the ventral crest of the thoracic vertebrae or, if present, from the ventral tips of the hypapophyses and the margin of the bony or membranous septum between them (Figs. 7a, b, 16a–h, 17a–h). This lung aponeurosis then passes, together with the inferior surface of the lung, to the lateral thoracic wall, where it fastens to the ribs, or passes over into the fascia endothoracica, respectively. There the lung aponeurosis is attached directly beneath the inferior margin of the lung, so that it descends, corresponding to the latter's course, from the vertebral joint of the first cranial rib, obliquely to its deepest point just above the joints between second and third vertebral and sternal ribs (Figs. 7a, b, 16a–h, 17a–h). From there it ascends in a posterodorsal direction along the lateral thoracic wall and reaches a point which is usually situated a little behind and beneath the anterior margin of the ilium (Figs. 7a, b, 16a–h, 17a–h).

Since the medial origin of the lung septum passes in a slight ventral arch corresponding to the ventrally oriented arch of the vertebral column or to the median septum which is formed by the hypapophyses, the horizontal aponeurosis forms a membrane ascending forward and backward from the middle, which

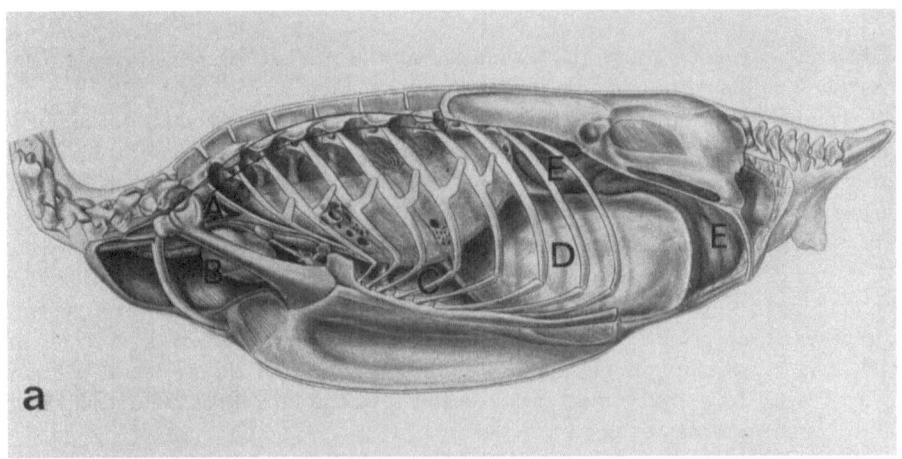

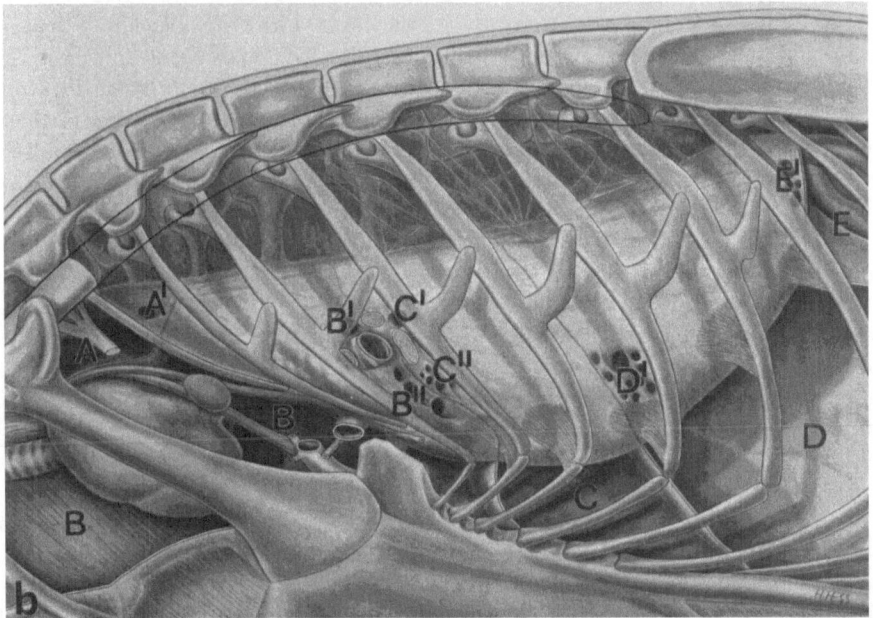

Fig. 7a and b. Drawing of a preparation of a northern mallard, *Anas platyrhynchos*, seen from lateral, left side. a) Demonstration of the horizontal and oblique septa. b) Separate demonstration of the cavum pulmonale. — Thoracic and abdominal wall have been removed except the ribs. The lung has been extirpated so that the cavum pulmonale is empty. Medially it is limited by the vertebral bodies with hypapophyses in the median septum, dorsolaterally by the transverse processes of the vertebrae and the vertebral ribs which incise far towards ventral. Ventrally the horizontal septum is stretched out which includes the penetrations for the primary bronchus and blood vessels at the lung hilus and the air sac ostia. The horizontal septum possesses the Mm. costopulmonales at its lateral attachment. Towards caudal it continues into the oblique septum. Beneath the horizontal septum lie the small cervical (*A*) and the large interclavicular (*B*) air sac which overlaps the shoulder girdle with coracoid and clavicle far cranially. Posteriorly anterior (*C*) and posterior thoracic (*D*) air sacs are situated. Medial to the oblique septum lies the abdominal air sac (*E*) above the viscera. The ostia (*A'*) for the cervical, (*B'*) for the interclavicular and (*C'*) for the anterior thoracic air sac as well as the additional ostia (*B''*) and (*C''*), the ostia (*D'*) for the posterior thoracic and (*E'*) for the abdominal air sac are found in the horizontal septum also ascends from the lateral attachments at the ribs and thoracic fascia to the vertebral column in a slightly dorsal direction (Figs. 7a, b, 16a–h, 17a–h).

The lung septa on both sides do not pass completely horizontal, but slightly sink towards both sides of the thorax, most markedly in the region of the middle of the lung, where they have both their deepest medial origin and their deepest insertion at the thoracic wall (Figs. 7a, b, 16a–h, 17a–h). The two septa do not always originate directly from the ventral tips of the vertebrae or hypapophyses. If the lungs are higher than the medial septum, as in herons and storks, or also in song birds, the medial septum may continue for a few millimeters in a ventral direction as a septum of the same qualities as the horizontal septa, so that, in this manner, the lung septa have a stalked origin from the vertebral column (Fig. 17a–h). However, course and attachment of the lung septa are not changed in any manner whatsoever.

Thus the horizontal septum of the lung is developed in the same position in all birds, from the penguins up to the song birds. In likewise constant manner the horizontal septa of the lung in all birds have small muscles, the Mm. costopulmonales, which originate, ventral to their lateral attachments, from the ribs and the adjoining regions of the fascia endothoracica. The first of these muscles originates from the first or second thoracic vertebral rib, near its inter-costal joint, or, as M. sternopulmonalis from the processus lateralis anterior of the sternum, partly passing more markedly from cranial to caudal (Figs. 7b, 11, 13, 15, 16a–h, 17a–h). The following muscles which usually are very well developed, originate in the region of the intercostal joints from the second and/or third rib pair, corresponding to the low level of the middle of the lung and the horizontal septum at this point. The last two, at the most three, Mm. costo-pulmonales originate from the adjoining vertebral ribs, always a little farther dorsally. These muscles, mostly 4 or 5 together, all originate a little ventral to the attachment of the horizontal septum, from the ribs and the neighbouring fascia, ascend, already fanning out, towards the septum and turn in the latter's direction, only to insert forming a variously wide fan (Figs. 7b, 11, 13, 15, 16a–h, 17a–h). At their origin they may already be so wide that they fuse into an uniform strip very soon, and thus form an uniform marginal zone of the horizontal septum, as in the rhea (Fig. 11). Generally, however, they form individual fans of muscle fibers separated from each other (Figs. 7b, 13, 15, 16a–h, 17a–h). Their total fiber length is, very constantly, about a third of the width of the horizontal septum in its middle and posterior part. The Mm. costopulmonales which are always existent in all species, may show more or less differences, specific to the species, in the thickness of their fiber layers and the width of the fanning. In the grey heron and common murre they are developed especially thin and weak.

The horizontal septum ventrally limits the dorsal part of the thoracic cavity, the cavum pulmonale (Huxley, 1882), that part which practically cannot experience any kind of diameter change because of the limited possibilities of mobility of the ribs. This cavity is totally occupied by the lungs; only occasionally a small amount of adipose tissue is found between septum and lung, for example between two large, superficial secondary bronchi or beneath the lateral margin of the lung. — The greatest depth of this cavity is in the region of the first or second intercostal joint, consequently very far cranially (Figs. 16a–h, 17a–h).

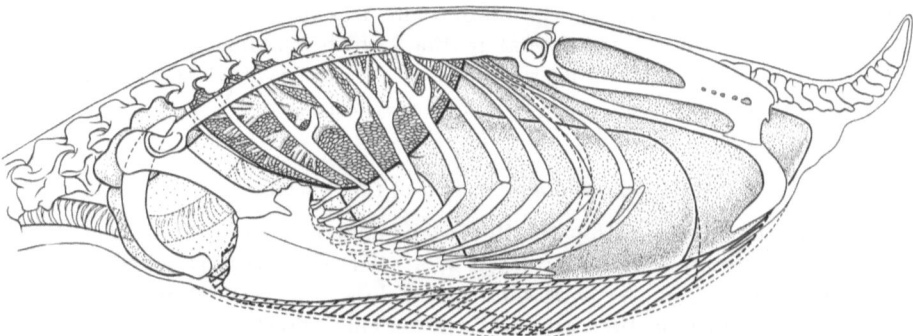

Fig. 8. Trunk of a mute swan, *Cygnus olor*, with outlines of the lung and the air sacs. Schematic demonstration of the positions that are occupied by the sternum together with the ribs against the vertebral column, during the respiratory motions. Solid lines: expiratory position. Dotted contours: deep inspiratory position in which the posterior air sacs are strikingly dilated

From there, in a caudal direction the dorsal thoracic cavity becomes continually more shallow. In the region of greatest depth the horizontal septum is connected to the pericardium (Figs. 16 a–h, 17 a–h). Here, coming from mediocranial between pericardium and septum, the primary bronchus enters the lung (Figs. 7 a, b, 13, 15, 16 a–h, 17 a–h). Cranial and further lateral to the primary bronchus, the pulmonal artery passes into the lung hilus, while the pulmonal vein leaves the lung caudal and medial to the primary bronchus and passes directly into the pericardium lying underneath (Figs. 13, 15).

Medial to the lung hilus the horizontal septum is also penetrated by the ostia of the interclavicular and the anterior thoracic air sac. Lateral to the lung hilus two additional, variously large ostia into these two air sacs are found (Figs. 7 a, b, 11, 13, 15). The horizontal septum is less markedly developed in the region of the lung hilus with its air sac ostia and the connection to the pericardium. In this anterior region, often near the lung tip, the ostium into the cervical air sac is situated. Caudal to the lung hilus, the horizontal septum possesses the great ostium into the posterior thoracic air sac at its lateral margin which is situated about midway between lung hilus and posterior end of the lung (Figs. 7 a, b, 11, 13, 15, 16 a–h, 17 a–h). In song birds this ostium is subdivided into a medial and an additional lateral ostium.

At the transversely situated posterior margin of the lung the horizontal septum splits in two membranes. The better developed membrane of the two turns ventrally, in a sharp curve and from there takes its course as oblique septum of the air sacs, while the second, weaker membrane turns dorsally, separates the lung from the cranial portion of the opisthonephros and attaches to the dorsal thoracic wall. This second, dorsal sheet of the horizontal septum is penetrated in its lateral part by the great ostium of the abdominal air sac (Figs. 7 a, b, 11, 16 a–h, 17 a–h).

It is characteristic that the Mm. costopulmonales, in the course of their insertions into the horizontal septum, spread around all lateral ostia, and, consequently, are parts of the cranial and caudal margins of the ostia. This is especially marked for the ostia into the posterior thoracic and the abdominal air sac (Figs. 7a, b, 15). Except the lateral portion, which contains the muscles, the horizontal septum is so thin that the underlying structures of the lung can transparently be seen. However, it is very coarse and resistant.

II. The Oblique Septum of the Air Sacs

The oblique septum within the thoracoabdominal cavity of the birds, which separates the majority of the large air sacs from the viscera is a continuation of the posterior end of the horizontal septum in a ventrocaudal direction, and, in its whole anterior portion, also in a ventrocranial direction. Thus the oblique septum, developed as a solid aponeurosis, limits a cavity which considerably unfolds ventral to the lungs, the cavum subpulmonale (Huxley, 1882). It is limited by the thoracic wall laterally and anteriorly, by the horizontal septum of the lung dorsally and medially in its anterior portion by the pericardium, in the large following portion by the oblique septum (Figs. 11, 13, 15).

At the lateral thoracic wall the oblique septum continues the lateral attachment of the horizontal septum, from which it has originated at the posterior margin of the lung. This lateral line of attachment passes laterally parallel to the vertebral column, underneath the bony pelvis as far as more or less distant behind the hip joint, after it had ascended together with the horizontal septum closely under the anterior margin of the ilium at the posterior lung pole (Figs. 7a, b, 13, 15, 16a–h, 17a–h). In the extension of its caudal attachment it shows close connections to the caudal extension of the ribs. The oblique septum with its dorsal attachment always extends 2 or 3 intercostal widths farther caudally than the last rib (in the plane of the intercostal joints) (Figs. 5a–c, 6a–c, 7a, 16a–h, 17a–h).

Then, the line of attachment of the oblique septum turns ventrally in a wide or narrow curve and passes towards the posterolateral margin of the sternum, forming a caudal prolongation of the lateral sternal margin. This ventral attachment of the oblique septum may take a variable course in different species, partly lateral and above the lateral sternal margin, partly further ventral and covered by the sternum. For once this depends on the extension of the caudal sternum, whether it projects far laterally with its processes or remains narrow. On the other hand the attachment of the oblique septum mostly is shifted in a ventromedial direction in different species, especially at the posterior sternal margin (Fig. 9), thus in ducks, and especially in the grey heron and coot.

The oblique septum, in its caudal portion, consequently forms a recess behind the end of the lung, which is limited laterally by the trunk wall and medially by the oblique septum. Because of the constant relation of its extension to the existence of caudal ribs, the form of the recess is characteristic for terrestrial and swimming types. As a consequence of the small caudal rib extension of the terrestrial form and its great angle between vertebral column and sternum, this recess is short but very wide (Figs. 6a–c, 17a–h), while it is developed shallower and longer in the swimming form (Figs. 5a–c, 7a, 16a–h). In penguins and auks, in which the ribs almost reach the caudal end of the abdominal cavity, the ribs may, contrary to most other species, extend as far as to the end of this

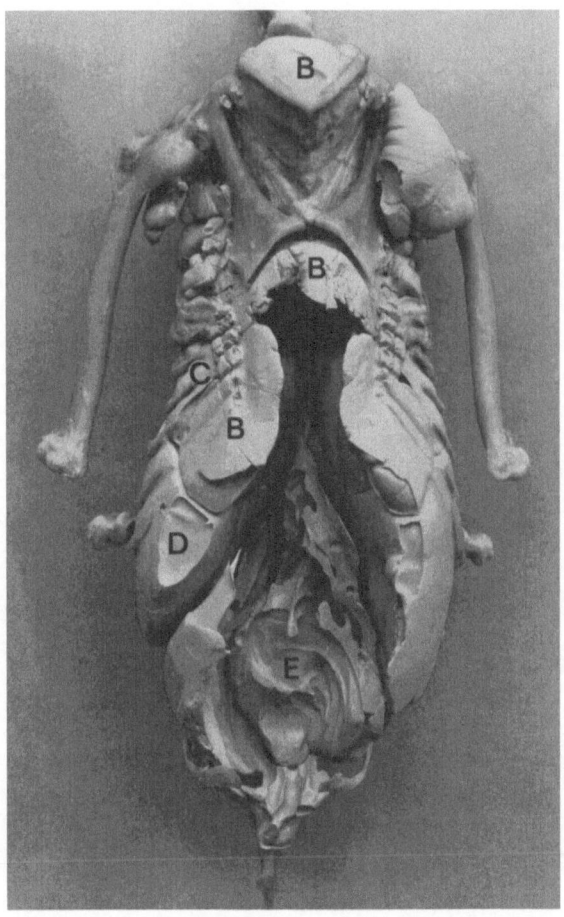

Fig. 9. Skeleton lung air sac preparation of a northern mallard, *Anas platyrhynchos*, seen from ventral. Sternum and sternal ribs have been removed. Coracoids and clavicles enclose the interclavicular air sac (*B*) which reaches far caudally with its lateral diverticula. Anterior (*C*) and posterior (*D*) thoracic air sac are medially limited by the oblique septum. The abdominal air sacs (*E*) show the impressions of the intestinal tract. ×0.6

recess or even overlap its inferior margin (Fig. 1). — The course of septal attachment, which is more lateral or more medial to the sternal margin, reaches a point near the anterior end of the sternal margin, shortly behind the articulation with the coracoid and variously far under the deepest lateral extension of the lung. From this point the oblique septum ascends dorsally and attaches to the pericardium medially, totally fusing with it laterally (Figs. 11, 12, 14).

The oblique septum first takes a transverse course, dorsally at its origin from the horizontal septum at the posterior margin of the lung, then in its lateral and ventral portion turns in a caudal direction, limiting the caudal recess of the cavum pulmonale in its course which is almost parallel to the body wall. Towards the vertebral column the oblique septum immediately turns from a

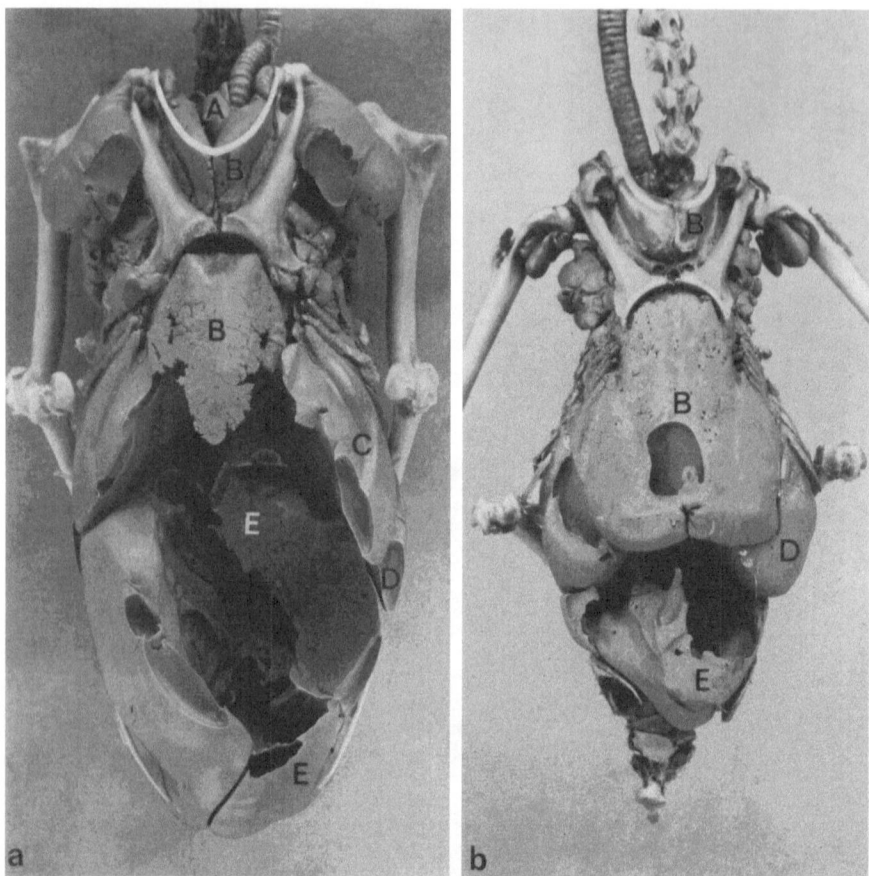

Fig. 10a and b. Skeleton lung air sac preparation seen from ventral, sternum and sternal ribs removed. Coracoids and clavicles enclose the interclavicular air sac (*B*). a) Domestic pigeon, *Columba domestica*. Median impar diverticulum of the interclavicular air sac between sternum and visceral bulk. Penetrating tissue bridges may be recognized. Large anterior (*C*) and small posterior (*D*) thoracic air sacs. Large abdominal (*E*) air sacs with impressions of the viscera. ×0.9. b) Jackdaw, *Corvus monedula*. Impar median diverticulum of the interclavicular air sac (*B*), very large with tissue bridges passing through it. Large posterior thoracic (*D*) and abdominal (*E*) air sacs, the latter with impressions of the viscera. ×0.9

transverse into a craniocaudal direction, namely at the ventral midline of the vertebral column or at the hypapophyses, respectively (Figs. 11, 13, 15). From this dorsal, twofold bent line of origin the septum passes obliquely in a ventro-lateral direction, to its inferior line of attachment and thus becomes a stretched plate, slightly bulging outward (Figs. 11, 12, 14). Cranially, the oblique septum fastens dorsal to the pericardium and fuses with it (Figs. 11, 16a–h, 17a–h). It cannot be decided unobjectionably, whether the oblique septum extends between the pericardial and septal wall on one hand and the thoracic wall on the other hand which are very close to each other, and whether it consequently forms the anterior boundary of the posterior cavity, or whether the subdivision in this region is brought about only by the walls of the interclavicular and anterior thoracic air sac, which are adjacent to each other. Taken the latter case, the oblique septum would issue into the lateral pericardial wall.

In the dorsal angle of the oblique septum, which is formed by the portion affixed transversely to the posterior lung margin and the portion affixed longitudinally to the thoracic vertebral column, a widely fanned muscle can always be found. Mostly, this muscle originates directly from the last or the two last hypapophyses. In some species the oblique septum originates as aponeurosis from the hypapophyses and not until 1–3 mm ventral to the origin the incorporation of muscles into the septum begins, as in ducks for example. In the rhea and in some ducks this muscle has a very wide extension at its origin already (Figs. 11, 12, 16a–h). It always extends fanlike in a ventral direction and in most species almost forms a semicircle, which accompanies the curvature of the oblique septum around its dorsal angle. The fiber length regularly is $^1/_5$ to $^1/_4$ of the total septal height. In its development this muscle, which I propose to call M. tensor septi obliqui, is similar to the Mm. costopulmonales. If they are weakly developed, it is also composed of only a thin fiber layer, and vice versa.

Solid muscle layers, which stem from the M. transversus abdominis of the abdominal wall, are found in the caudal end of the oblique septum in some species, however to a degree considerably varying individually. This can be very well observed in swans.

In the region of the caudal oblique septum, individual weaker or more marked muscle crests may project from the trunk wall, apparently vestigia of the ontogenetic extension of the caudal recess of the cavum subpulmonale, in the course of which the septum was broadened by the splitting of parts from the lateral trunk wall.

The oblique septum is attached to the following loci: dorsally to the vertebral column and the posterior septum, caudally to the lateral trunk wall, ventrally to the lateral trunk wall and the sternal margin and cranial within the pericardium. The attachment to the trunk wall is always caused by its issuing into the fascia endothoracica or transversalis. The oblique septum, together with the horizontal septum and the lateral trunk wall encloses the cavum subpulmonale (Huxley, 1882). This cavity beneath the lung is very wide dorsally and becomes increasingly narrower towards ventral, in cross section being bent like a comma towards medial (Figs. 16a–h, 17a–h). The cavum subpulmonale also becomes narrower within the caudal recess. This recess ends ventrally and caudally with rounded margins. It is totally occupied by the anterior and posterior thoracic air sacs. The oblique septa of both sides enclose the anterior portion of the visceral sac with the heart, thus forming the lateral and dorsal boundary of the cavum pericardioabdominale (Figs. 11, 12, 14, 16a–h, 17a–h).

Special relations are found in song birds, woodpeckers and swifts. In these species the ventral attachments of the oblique septa pass towards the posterolateral end of the sternum and are fastened to the posterior margin of the sternum (Fig. 14). Further cranially, the two oblique septa do not find any direct ventral attachment to the thoracic wall, but they fuse a little above the sternum and pass cranially into the ventral pericardial wall, as otherwise happens only laterally. The oblique septa thus on all sides enclose the content of the cranial abdominal cavity, liver and gizzard, similar to a bag that cranially issues into the peri-cardium. The functionally necessary attachment at the ventral abdominal wall is produced by narrow, very coarse tissue bridges, which span the cavity between the united oblique septa and the inside of the sternum. This cavity is developed as an air sac. These coarse tissue bridges are very numerous cranially between pericardium and the most anterior part of the oblique septa, towards caudal they become, less numerous, but can be demonstrated as individual connections as far as to the end of the sternum. This cavity, formed between the trunk wall and the oblique septa is occupied laterally by the two thoracic, ventrally however by the caudal portion of the interclavicular air sac (Figs. 10b, 14, 17a–h).

III. Position of the Viscera and Blood Vessels

Cranial to the lateral air sac cavity and in front of the pericardial cavity lies another large cavity within the thorax. This is the anterior part of the cavum subpulmonale of Huxley. Dorsally it is limited by the vertebral column and especially by the ventral cervical musculature, which originates from the last cervical and first thoracic vertebrae, more precisely, from the often present hypapophyses, which in some species are split like a T on their ventral side. Dorsolaterally, the horizontal septum above the anterior lung portion follows. The lateral wall is formed by the anterior ribs, the coracoid, the clavicle and the membrana coracoclavicularis, which ventrally fuse with the sternum. Cranially the cavity is covered only by the M. constrictor colli and the skin. The inter-clavicular air sac and the two small cervical air sacs are situated in this anterior cavum subpulmonale.

A large number of structures passes through the space of the interclavicular and cervical air sac. Trachea and esophagus enter from cranial. The trachea, shortly after its entrance or not until just before the lung hilus, is split in the two primary bronchi (Figs. 13, 15, 19b). In most birds the bifurcation is complicatedly structured by the development of the syrinx, muscles pass from the thoracic wall to the trachea and/or syrinx. Besides, vessels and nerves for the wings and the neck, pass through this space.

In deglutitional birds like fish catching species, the gate which is formed by the two primary bronchi and the ventral lung surface and through which the esophagus passes, is always very wide. It is narrow in grain eating species having a crop. The esophagus passes between pericardium and vertebral column and at first is enclosed on both sides by the oblique septum (Figs. 16a–h, 17a–h). If the esophagus does not dilate very much, the two oblique septa in their cranial portion may fuse dorsal and ventral to the esophagus and thus enclose it. If the esophagus must be passed by great boli, however, it is freely suspended between the septa by a dorsal mesentery. Dorsal to the esophagus the aorta is always rigidly embedded directly ventral to the vertebral column, in the common basis of the horizontal and oblique septa (Figs. 16a–h, 17a–h). If the horizontal septa have a stalked origin, the aorta lies in the septum between the lungs, from which the horizontal septa originate.

The space, which is limited laterally by the oblique septa, dorsally by the pelvis and ventrally by the sternum and the inferior abdominal wall, the cavum cardioabdominale, contains the rest of the viscera. In the anterior portion of this space, about as far as it is covered by the sternum, lies the large liver. Ventromedially, for its whole length it is affixed to the sternum by a mesentery. Cranially, at the right, is the vessel connection to the heart, dorsally to the aorta and caudally to the right kidney (renal portal system), and to the intestinal tract. A membrane originates from the dorsal mesentery of the liver towards both sides, connecting to the pericardium cranially, laterally to the oblique septa (Figs. 11, 16a–h, 17a–h) and caudally to the ventral abdominal wall, variably far behind the caudal sternal margin. This membrane is the posthepatic septum (Poole, 1909; Ede, 1964) by which the liver is separated and therefore lies in a special compartment of the abdominal cavity. This septum is extremely thin in song birds. Dorsal and caudal to this membrane lies the gall bladder, and stretched between the two mesenteries the esophagus which converts into the proventriculus and then into the gizzard. The gizzard in variable extension grows together with the left septum posthepaticum which is lying on its ventral surface. By this the gizzard is affixed to the left oblique septum (Figs. 16a–h, 17a–h).

In the posterior part of the abdominal cavity the intestinal loops in their convolutions specific to the species are situated, freely mobile and attached and supplied only by the dorsal mesentery. Kidneys, adrenal glands, gonads and their efferent pathes are directly grown together with the dorsal abdominal wall or, as the oviduct, possess a mesentery of their own. The intestinal convolutions normally do not quite fill the whole posterior abdominal cavity. They are situated on the ventral abdominal wall, suspended from their dorsal mesentery. The remaining space is occupied by the abdominal air sacs (Figs. 16a–h, 17a–h).

The body cavity of birds is subdivided into the following compartments with specific contents each: dorsally, in the thoracic region, the horizontal septa confine the lung cavities. Ventral to the lungs, cranially in the region of the shoulder girdle, lies the cavity of the cervical and interclavicular air sacs, through which pass trachea and primary bronchi, esophagus, numerous vessels and many nerves. Adjoining is the pericardial cavity with its immediate connection to the lung hilus. Ventral to the lungs, medially limited by the oblique septa, the cavities for the anterior and posterior thoracic air sacs follow, which extend as far as lateral beneath the hip joint. The anterior portion of the abdominal cavity, lying between the oblique septa and ventral to the lungs, which adjoins directly to the pericardium from dorsal, contains liver, esophagus and gizzard. Because of a horizontal membrane development the liver lies in a ventroanterior compartment of the abdomen of its own. The space for the gizzard situated dorsally to the latter, which is also fixed laterally by the liver membrane, opens into the wide posterior abdominal cavity behind the caudal lung margin. It contains the urogenital organs, grown together dorsally, and the intestinal convolutions freely mobile because they are suspended by a dorsal mesentery only. Therefore a large amount of space is available for the abdominal air sacs in this portion of the body cavity.

Extension and Position of the Air Sacs

The extension of the air sacs and the diverticula originating from them varies considerably in the different species. The most simple relations are shown in

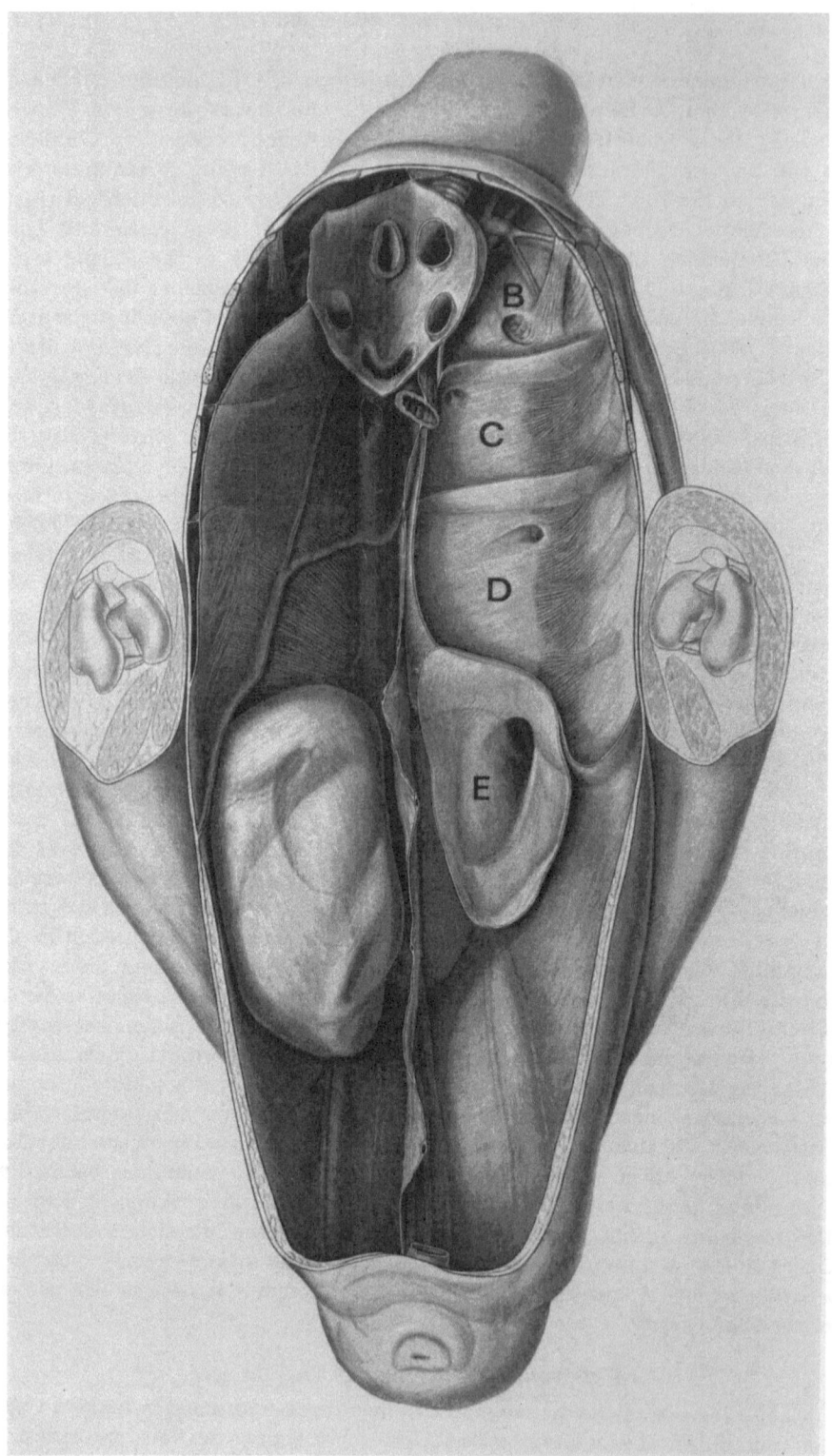

Fig. 11

the diving species and those swimming under water, penguins, cormorants, loons, grebes, auks and diving ducks. They possess nine well developed, large air sacs: two cervical, one interclavicular, and two of each anterior thoracic, posterior thoracic and abdominal air sacs, additionally a few small diverticula around the shoulder joint and along the cervical vertebral column (Figs. 1, 5a, b).

Other appendages of the air sac system are found only in the terrestrial or the water birds only swimming, developed best in the large, well flying species like swans, storks and herons, buzzards and large song birds. Large parts of the skeleton are pneumatised by air sac diverticula in these species, additionally, large diverticula are extended between the urogenital organs and the dorsal trunk wall, between the pelvic and cervical musculature, accompanying central vascular and nerve bundles. These systems of air sac diverticula vary from species to species and are not to be discussed at this point. The birds use air as construction material for a diminution of their specific gravity. These diverticula do not play any part in the avian respiration (Duncker, 1968b). In the following discussion only the nine large air sacs will be considered and demonstrated.

I. The Cervical and the Impar Interclavicular Air Sacs

These air sacs occupy the cranial thoracic cavity which is situated beneath the inferior cervical region and the cranial thoracic vertebral column and under the anterior lung portions, and which is limited laterally and ventrally by the clavicles, the coracoids, the membrana coracoclavicularis and the anterior thoracic wall with ribs and sternum (Figs. 1, 2, 5a–c, 6a–c, 7a, b, 9, 10a, b). The cervical air sacs on both sides originate from their ostium out of the first ventrobronchus in the anterior half of the lungs, which also can be shifted far towards the lung tip (Figs. 20c, 28a, b, 29a–c). The impar interclavicular air sac on both sides obtains its main ostium from the third ventrobronchus directly at the lung hilus, a little medial and cranial to the hilus (Figs. 20b, c, 28a, b, 29a–c). Besides, the interclavicular air sac has an additional ostium from each lung, lateral to the lung hilus, which mostly is situated at the lung margin, namely at its deepest and furthest ventral point (Figs. 19b, 21c, 22c, 28a, b, 29a–c). The ostium is of variable size and unlike the other ostia, it does not directly lead into a lateral

Fig. 11. Drawing of a preparation of the American rhea, *Rhea americana*, seen from ventral. Ventral abdominal wall removed, whole intestinal tract and the heart extirpated. On the right side of the preparation the oblique septum is demonstrated, the ventral margin of which has been cut off. It passes into the pericardium cranially and on its surface it contains the line of attachment of the post-hepatic septum. In front of it, the pars affixa hepatis can be seen. In the dorsal part of the oblique septum passes the V. cava inferior. In the caudal part of the septum the M. tensor septi obliqui can be recognized which is partly covered by the abdominal air sac which bulges deep into the abdominal cavity. — On the left side of the preparation the oblique septum and the wall of the abdominal air sac have largely been removed. Thus the cavum subpulmonale and the horizontal septum may be seen. The septa between the anteriorly situated interclavicular (*B*) and anterior thoracic (*C*) air sacs as well as between anterior and posterior (*D*) thoracic air sacs, can be recognized, besides also the ostia into these and into the abdominal air sac (*E*). In the lateral marginal portion of the horizontal septum the Mm. costopulmonales are broadly developed

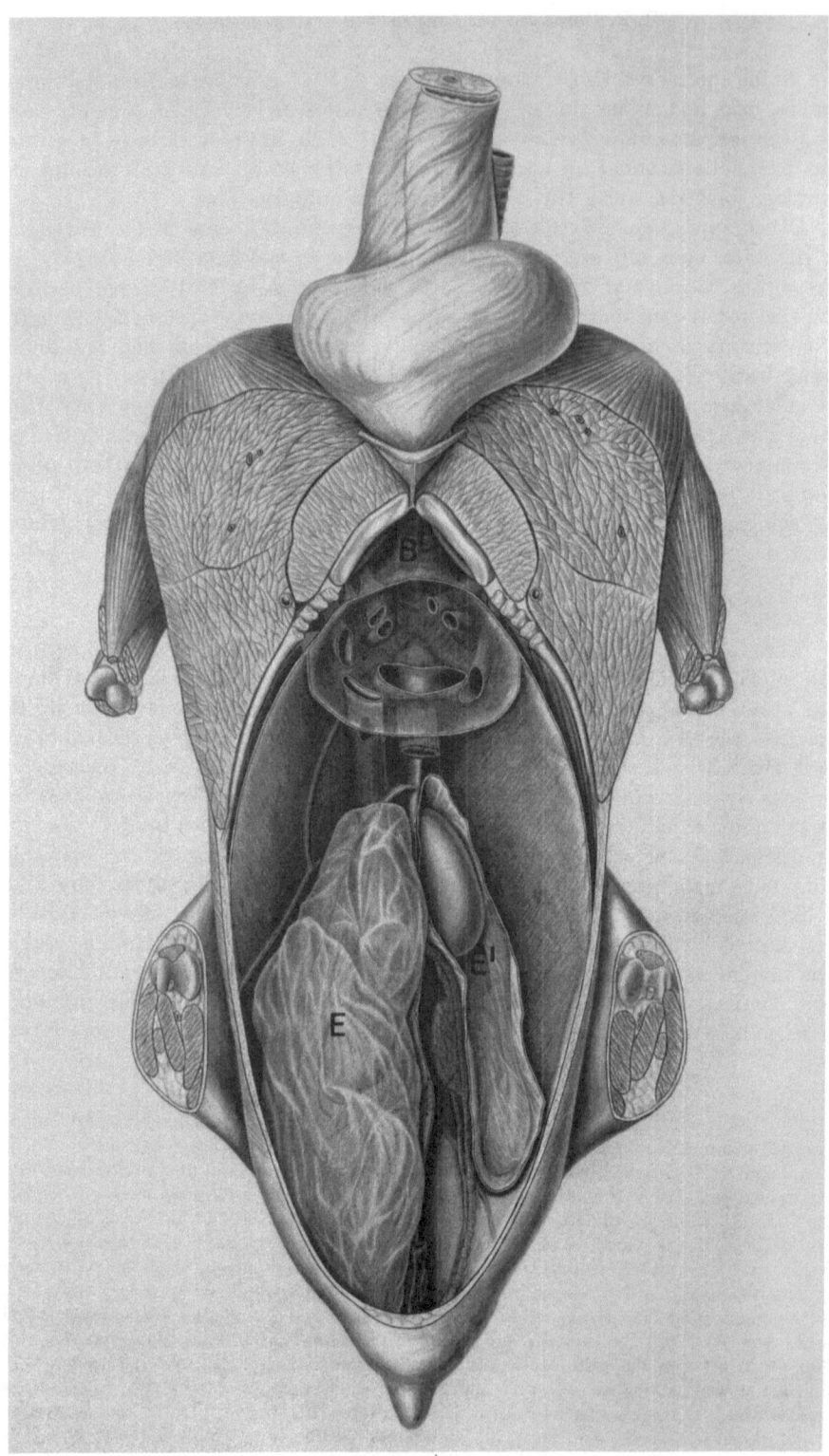

Fig. 12. (Legend see p. 48)

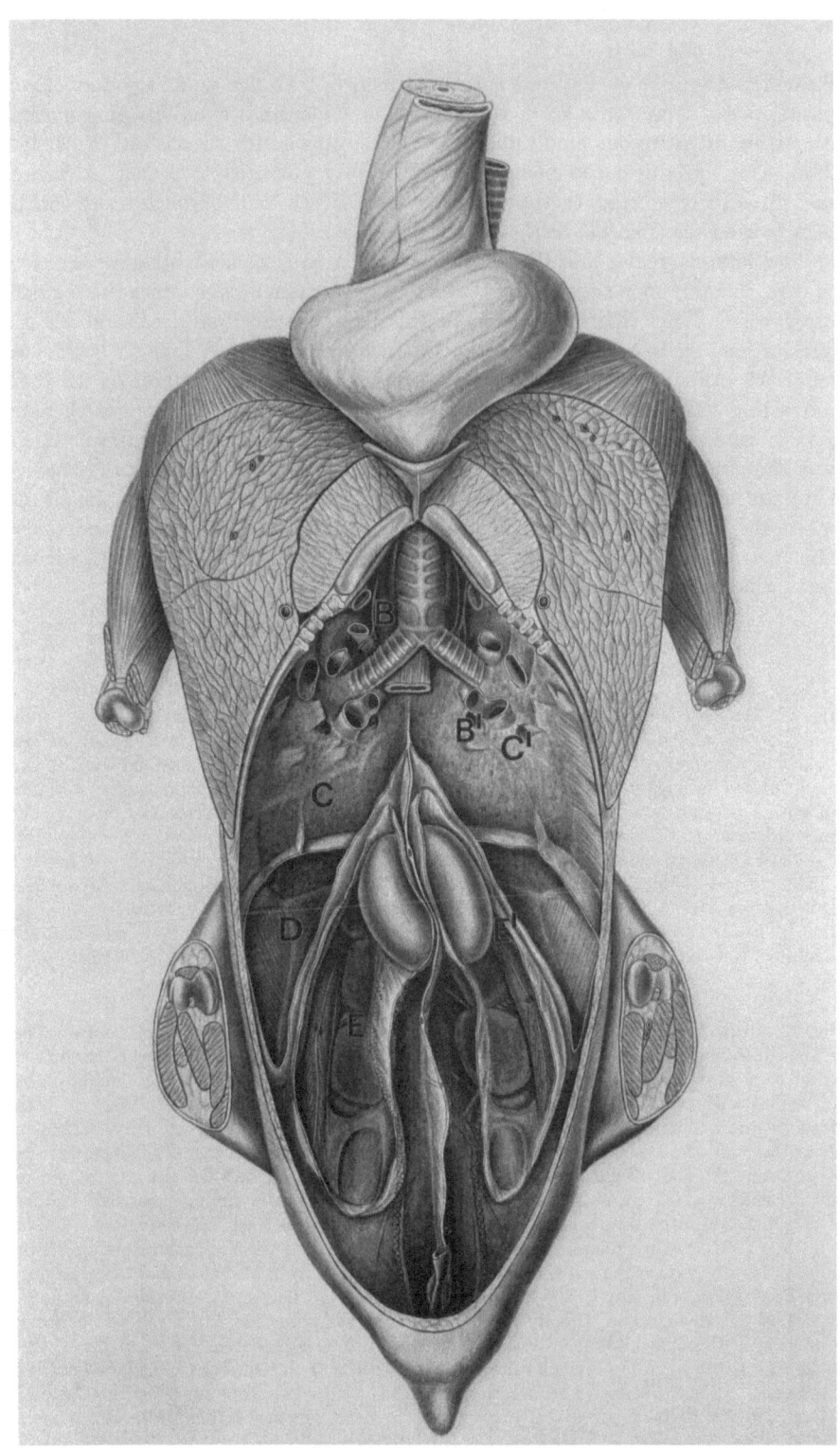

Fig. 13. (Legend see p. 48)

branch of the first or second ventrobronchus, but at this point the network of parabronchi, originating from the ostium, or sometimes even the lung surface consisting of numerous small delicate vesicles, opens into the air sac (Figs. 21c, 22c). This variably sized opening is only rarely gathered to a short bronchus and directly connected to the lateral branch of the ventrobronchus, as can be seen in the rhea (Fig. 11) or the stork.

The interclavicular and the cervical air sacs originate, as all other air sacs too, as thin, membranous sacs at their ostia and with their walls contact those structures which limit their extension, in this case the horizontal septum on the inferior lung surface and the anterior thoracic wall. These air sacs on both sides join each other in a horizontal plane, forming a dividing membrane with their contacting walls. A large number of vessels pass through the cranial thoracic cavity, additionally nerves, esophagus, trachea with syrinx, primary bronchi and the muscles passing towards them (Figs. 7a, b, 11, 13, 15, 16a–h, 17a–h). They are surrounded by the air sacs, so that they pass freely through the air sac space and are braced by a thin membrane, usually towards one wall side only. The membrane is formed by the growing together of the walls of both air sac parts which surround the vessel.

Fig. 12. Drawing of a preparation of the domestic pigeon, *Columba domestica*, seen from ventral. Ventral abdominal wall and sternum which has been disarticulated at the ribs and coracoids, are removed, the whole intestinal tract extirpated, the pericardium opened and the heart has been cut off at its vascular connections. The oblique septum ventrally continues on both sides into the pericardium, its ventral attachment to the sternal margin has been removed together with the sternum. In front of and lateral to the pericardium lies the interclavicular air sac (*B*). On the right side of the preparation the attachment of the post-hepatic septum to the oblique septum can be seen. In the cavum cardioabdominale the two thin walled, large abdominal air sacs (*E*) are situated. The left of the two has been opened so that its ostium (*E'*) and the left testis, which bulges deep into its cavity from dorsal are exhibited. Between the two abdominal air sacs lies the cut margin of the intestinal mesentery, anteriorly, beneath the pericardium the esophagus is cut

Fig. 13. Drawing of the preparation of Fig. 12, domestic pigeon, seen from ventral. The pericardium and the oblique septa have been removed on both sides, the cut margins of which may be recognized in front of the two opened abdominal air sacs (*E*). Thereby, the horizontal septum and the inferior lung surface with the lung hilus are exhibited on both sides. In the abdominal air sacs the markedly bulging testes are lying cranially, caudal to them these air sacs are attached to the ventral surface of the kidneys. (*E'*) demarcates the ostium into the abdominal air sac. Between the abdominal air sacs lies the cut margin of the mesentery which cranially fuses with the oblique septa to a common, median septum of origin. Beneath the bifurcation of the trachea the esophagus is cut off, before the primary bronchus lies the A. pulmonalis in the lung hilus, lateral to it the V. jugularis, on the right side of the preparation the cut off aortic arc is situated in front of and medial to the A. pulmonalis. Further cranially, in the interclavicular air sac (*B*) lie the Aa. carotides communes, lateral to the trachea and directly at the margin of the coracoids. Caudal to the primary bronchus, in the lung hilus lies the V. pulmonalis with two branches, and medial to it the ostium (*B'*) into the interclavicular air sac (*B*), lateral to it the ostium (*C'*) into the anterior thoracic (*C*) air sac. Between both air sacs the wall is reduced to a few tissue bridges. Lateral in the anterior thoracic air sac (*C*) are the Mm. costopulmonales. The posterior thoracic air sac (*D*) is relatively small

The two cervical air sacs meet ventral to the vertebral column and its musculature and grasp the esophagus between. However, they always reach only as far as to the lateral midline of the esophagus, there they meet the dorsal parts of the interclavicular air sac, forming a horizontally dividing membrane. This membrane passes very regularly from the lateral midline of the esophagus to the lateral wall of the anterior thoracic cavity (Figs. 16a–h, 17a–h). Ventral to this membrane the portions of the interclavicular air sac in a similar manner enclose the ventral part of the esophagus and the trachea. Ventral to the trachea the dividing membrane between the opposite parts of the interclavicular air sac is always diminished, usually across the whole anterior wall of the sac as far as the pericardium. Because of this regular and wide communication the interclavicular air sac is impar (Figs. 16a–h, 17a–h).

In large birds the opposite walls of the cervical air sacs grow together to form a mesoesophageum between the vertebral column and the esophagus. In corresponding manner, the dorsal portions of the interclavicular air sac form a mesotracheale between esophagus and trachea (Fig. 16a–h). The cervical air sacs and the dorsal portions of the interclavicular sac always incorporate the great vascular-nerve bundle of the inferior neck into their separating membranes. Within this membrane, following structures, as far as they are developed symmetrically, are found: nervus vagus, vena jugularis and arteria carotis. The carotic artery in its course through the membrane between the two air sacs, is accompanied on both sides by a glandula thyreoidea as well as one or two glandulae parathyreoideae.

The Aa. subclaviae usually protrude more markedly into the interclavicular air sac, the membrane, fastened to the arteries, passes towards dorsal and lateral. The one or two pairs of muscles which pass from the trachea, the syrinx or the primary bronchi towards the anterior thoracic wall, are surrounded by the air sac on all sides, so that they pass through the interclavicular air sac, free of any membranous fastenings. Caudally, the interclavicular air sac in its dorsal portion ends at the anterior pericardial wall, and at the great vascular trunks of the heart directly in front of the hilus of the lung, where its main ostium is situated, too.

If the cervical air sacs are well developed, they reach caudally as far as near the hilus of the lung and cranially may overlap the clavicle beneath the cervical musculature (Figs. 4c, 5a, c, 6b). Their separating membrane against the interclavicular air sac then passes horizontally towards the anterior lateral thoracic wall. However, cervical air sacs of this size are only present in penguins, swans, ducks, geese, falcons and buzzards. In the majority of the well flying species, the interclavicular air sac instead expands and fills the anterior space. The cervical air sacs then become shorter both cranially and caudally, and their separating membrane against the interclavicular air sac does not pass lateral to the thoracic wall anymore, but in a dorsal direction towards the vertebral column, as in storks, herons, fowllike and song birds, in which the cervical sacs become very small (Fig. 4a, b). They are present in almost all birds and their separating membrane against the interclavicular air sac generally maintains its relation to the vessels and nerves. If the cervical sacs become very small, the vessels and nerves shift from lateral to the esophagus. In the material studied, cervical air sacs are lacking only in loons and grebes.

Large cervical air sacs push their way between anterior scapula and superior coracoid on one hand and anterosuperior thoracic wall on the other hand (Fig. 4c). If the cervical air sacs become smaller the dorsal parts of the interclavicular air sac take over their position (Fig. 4a, b). These three air sacs thus form a unity which may be viewed as a functional entity.

Individually, it is dependent on the structure of the anterior thorax, the presence and size of a crop and probably also the analogous type of construction of the particular species, for instance in diving birds, how far these air sacs fill the anterior thoracic cavity and even overlap the clavicula cranially (Figs. 1, 2, 5a–c, 6a–c). Furthermore, in all three air sacs small septa may protrude from the walls in a very variable manner and more or less subdivide the sacs without a substantial change of the fundamental relations.

Regularly, diverticula pass from the cervical air sacs to the cervical vertebral column, which, generally along the vertebral vessels, issue into a cranial direction, pneumatise the vertebral bodies and penetrate into the epidural space of the vertebral canal. Series of diverticula invade the cervical musculature and accompany the branches of the plexus brachialis. Their extension varies from species to species. In some species the separating membrane is incomplete, allowing a fusion of the opposite cervical sacs above the esophagus, for instance in chickens. In loons and grebes all the diverticula originating from the cervical air sacs are lacking.

The interclavicular air sac gives off diverticula around the shoulder joint and between the muscles originating there; from there also into the humerus, furthermore into the sternum, into the coracoids and into the clavicles, additionally often an impar diverticulum — variously well developed — through the space between the primary bronchi towards caudal between esophagus and pericardium. As already mentioned above, these diverticula are almost completely lacking in diving species.

In large birds like swans, storks, cranes and in all song birds, the interclavicular air sac extends as far as into the space between pericardium and sternum, and penetrates caudally along the whole width of the sternum, generally overlapping the heart tip (Figs. 9, 10a, 16a–c); in song birds the interclavicular sac regularly reaches the caudal end of the sternum (Figs. 10b, 14, 17a–c). This enlargement of the interclavicular air sac is, contrary to all other large air sacs, not developed as an uniform space, but penetrated by a large number of mostly narrow yet coarse tissue bridges, which connect the pericardium with the internal surface of the sternum, especially with the anterior and lateral sternal margin (Figs. 9, 10a, b, 14, 16a–h, 17a–h). The tissue bridges continue as far as to the posterior sternal margin distributed loosely, however. Their function is apparent: they are to give the oblique septum, partly directly, mostly via the pericardium a solid attachment to the sternum especially at the cranial sternal portion. Thus this part of the interclavicular air sac is very similar to a pneumatised spongy bone. Since this portion of the interclavicular air sac originates from its impar, ventromedially situated portion, it is just as uniform and not divided in a right and a left portion.

The interclavicular and the two cervical air sacs basically differ from the rest of the great air sacs in that way, that a number of structures, like trachea and primary bronchi, esophagus and muscles, vessels, and nerves pass freely through the air sac space, generally suspended by a thin membrane, similar to a meso from one side of the wall. Additionally, their wall is divided by protruding septa. At these points where the interclavicular air sac penetrates into the region between pericardium and sternum, the space formed is always bridged by a large number of narrow yet very coarse tissue bridges, so that both walls of this space are held at a constant distance from each other and that thereby the oblique septa are attached ventrocranially via the pericardium.

II. The Anterior and Posterior Thoracic Air Sacs

These two thoracic air sacs are regularly developed as pairs. The space which they occupy is relatively smoothly limited. They lie under the posterior part of the horizontal septum, from the lung hilus as far as to the caudal lung margin, extending along the whole width of this septum. The medial wall is formed by the oblique septum, in its total extension, the lateral wall by the lateral thoracic and abdominal wall (Figs. 13, 15). Cranially, the space between the oblique septum and the pericardium, respectively, and thoracic wall, is limited by the vessels passing to the wings (Fig. 7a, b). In large birds, a membrane formed by the adjacent walls of the anterior thoracic and the interclavicular air sac, is the limitation, especially directly beneath the horizontal septum (Fig. 11). In th eanterior thoracic portion the space for these air sacs is wide dorsally and becomes narrower, like a wedge, towards ventral, corresponding to the curvature of the body wall (Figs. 7a, b, 9, 10a, b, 11, 12–15, 16a–h, 17a–h). In the posterior abdominal portion this space has become very narrow dorsally and issues into a sharp ventral and dorsal edge (Figs. 16a–h, 17a–h). In relation to the caudal extension of the ribs and thereby in relation to the form of the body, the space of the thoracic air sacs is long in swimming species and gains little height towards caudal (Figs. 1, 5a–c, 7a, 9). In the terrestrial form, on the contrary, it is almost completely wedge-shaped, with the tip behind the lung hilus and is limited caudally by a large curvature (Figs. 2, 6a–c, 10a, b).

Special relations are found in song birds. Due to the extension of the interclavicular air sac between pericardium and sternum as far as its caudal end, the attachment of the oblique septum has been shifted so far ventromedially on both sides, that in these species the opposite oblique septa attach and grow together ventrally, and are connected to the sternum by only a few coarse tissue bridges (Figs. 10b, 14, 17a–h). The posterior thoracic air sacs — the anterior thoracic air sacs are united with the interclavicular sac in singing birds — and the posterior part of the interclavicular sac now enclose the medial visceral sac which is surrounded by the oblique septa (Figs. 10b, 14, 17a–h). The posterior thoracic air sacs are separated from the posterior portion of the interclavicular air sac not by the oblique septa but only by their adjacent walls, forming a membrane which in all other birds has its place at that point at which the oblique septum inserts ventrally (Figs. 10b, 14, 17a–h).

The anterior thoracic air sac originates from its main ostium out of the third ventrobronchus, medial and a little caudal to the lung hilus (Figs. 11, 13, 19b,

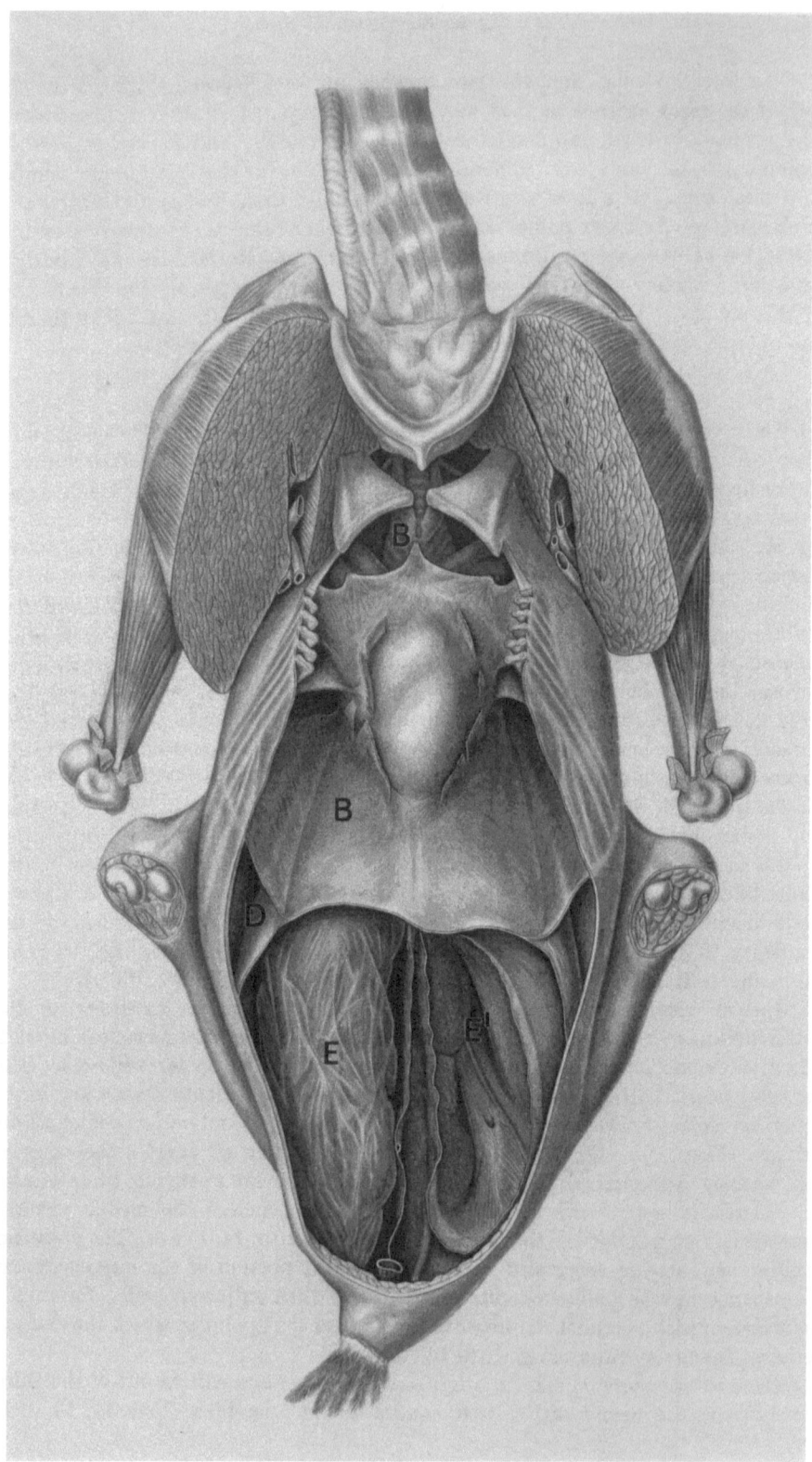

Fig. 14. (Legend see p. 54)

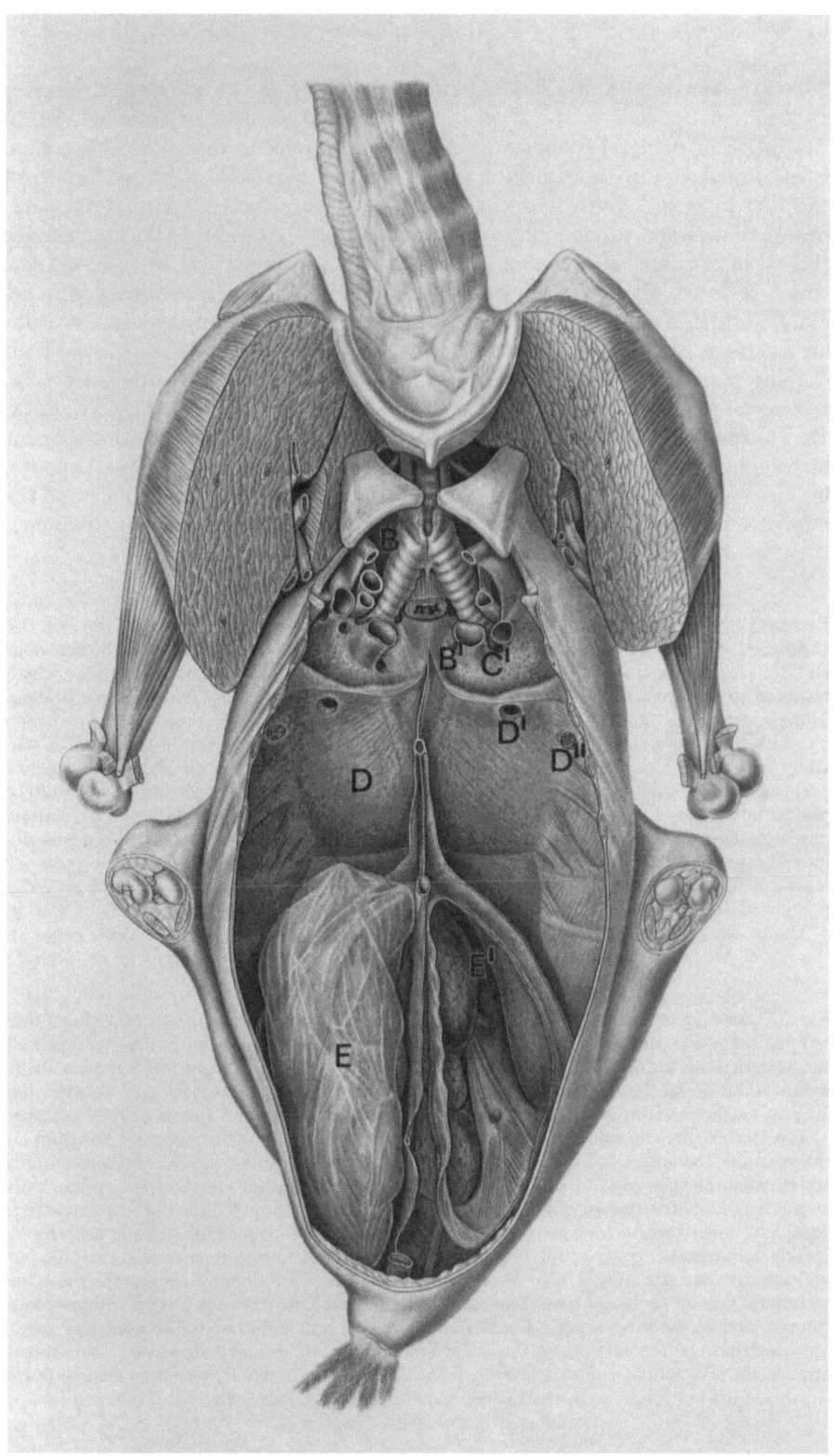

Fig. 15. (Legend see p. 54)

20c, 21c, 28a, b, 29a, b). The anterior thoracic air sac, in all species, receives an additional ostium at the front of the lung margin near its anterior wall, in the region of the largest thickness of the lung, lateral to the hilus. This ostium is of various size in the different species, and at this point a lateral branch of the first or second ventrobronchus opens into the air sac via the lateral parabronchial network, or via many small, communicating vesicles of the lung surface (Figs. 7b, 21c, 22c, 28a, b, 29a–c). In song birds, the anterior thoracic air sac, which is fused with the interclavicular air sac, also possesses this additional ostium, which is situated directly behind the lateral ostium for the interclavicular air sac (Figs. 22c, 29c).

The posterior thoracic air sac has its main ostium, which originates from a large laterobronchus, in the middle of the lateral lung margin (Figs. 7a, b, 11, 13, 15, 16a–h, 17a–h, 19b, 20c, 21c, 22c, 28a, b, 29a–c). The posterior thoracic air sac, besides the main ostium from the laterobronchus present in all species, in most species receives additional inflow from the parabronchial net of the lateroventral lung portion. Mostly, the laterobronchus opens up obliquely funnel-

Fig. 14. Drawing of a preparation of a carrion crow, *Corvus corone*, seen from ventral. Ventral abdominal wall removed together with the sternum which was disarticulated at the coracoids and the ribs. In the anterior portion of the preparation the pericardium is exhibited which attaches to the sternum via cranial and lateral partly considerably broad tissue bridges. The pericardium continues caudally and laterally into the oblique septa which have been united behind the pericardium and dorsal to the sternum, and thus form a closed plate ventrally which can be seen here. The united oblique septa are attached above the anterior pericardium and are caudally cut off at the posterior margin of the sternum. In front of the pericardium, lateral, ventral and caudal to it, lies the interclavicular air sac (*B*) with its impar median caudoventral recess which is so large developed in song birds and has laterally incorporated the anterior thoracic air sacs in these species. On both sides of the posterior margin of the oblique septa the posterior thoracic air sac (*D*) has been opened. In the posterior portion of the preparation the viscera have been removed, in the middle the cut margin of the mesentery is visible. On both sides lie the thin walled large abdominal air sacs (*E*), the left of which has been cut off along its dorsal line of attachment so that its ostium (*E'*) can be seen

Fig. 15. Drawing of the preparation of Fig. 14, carrion crow, seen from ventral. The united oblique septa and the pericardium have been removed so that the horizontal septum and the inferior lung surface with the lung hilus are exhibited. The oblique septa remain to be seen at their dorsal line of attachment, which pass together with the mesentery between the lungs towards cranial in order to fuse in a common dorsomedian root. Beneath the bifurcation of the trachea lies the cut off esophagus, lateral and in front of the primary bronchus in the region of the lung hilus the A. pulmonalis, the V. jugularis and the A. carotis communis are situated, on the right side additionally the aortic arc. Caudally to the primary bronchus in the lung hilus lies the V. pulmonalis, medial to it the ostium (*B'*) for the interclavicular, lateral to it the ostium (*C'*) for the anterior thoracic air sac which are fused in song birds. Clearly recognizable is the wall between anterior thoracic/interclavicular air sac (*B*) and the posterior thoracic air sac (*D*). Near this wall the posterior thoracic air sac has the large ostium (*D'*) out of the large laterobronchus in the middle between lung margin and vertebral column, and at the lung margin lies the additional ostium (*D''*) out of the accessory parabronchial net. In the margin of the horizontal septum lie the well developed Mm. costopulmonales. The left of the thin walled, large abdominal air sacs is cut off so that only its dorsal field of fusion with the kidney and the dorsal abdominal wall remains and its funnel-shaped ostium (*E'*) can be seen

shaped towards the lateral lung margin (Figs. 16 a–e, 17 c–e, 21 c, 22 c). The part
of the funnel-shaped opening which lies close to the lateral wall and is drawn
out long and wide, shows numerous small openings into the parabronchial net
of the lateral lung portion in swans and ducks, chickens and pigeons, a few
openings in storks and cormorants (Figs. 7 a, b, 16 d, e, 19 b, 21 c). In loons a
subdivision of this ostium into a large ostium out of the laterobronchus, situated
in the middle of the posteroinferior surface of the lung, and a mostly smaller
ostium out of the parabronchial net, situated at the lung margin, is indicated.
This division has been completed in song birds. They possess two ostia which
don't seem to have any relation to each other (Figs. 15, 17 d, e, 22 c, 29 c). In
penguins and emus not only an additional second ostium of the posterior thoracic
air sac is lacking but in these species the funnel-shaped opening of the laterobronchus also does not have any openings out of the parabronchi (Figs. 20 c, 28 a).

At the ostia, the thin air sac wall turns over to the horizontal septum and
continues its course on the oblique septum and the lateral trunk wall. Thus
the air sacs completely fill the space described above. On a transverse plane,
running from dorsal to ventral, the anterior and posterior thoracic air sacs
meet and with their adjacent walls form a membrane, which subdivides the
space in an anterior and a larger posterior portion (Figs. 7 a, b, 11, 13, 15).
This dividing membrane may be sloped a little more, so that it passes from
dorsocranial towards ventrocaudal, or forms a plane directed obliquely from
posteromedial towards anterolateral.

The position of the dividing membrane is subject to significant variations
as are form and size of the anterior air sac, which is generally considerably smaller
than the posterior thoracic air sac (Figs. 1, 2, 5 b, 6 a–c, 7 a, b, 11, 15). The anterior
thoracic air sac is present in all birds. Generally it is about $^1/_4$ the size of the
posterior thoracic air sac. Seldom it is bigger, as in swans and storks where it
is $^1/_3$ the size of the posterior thoracic air sac. In pigeons and fowllike birds on
the other hand the anterior thoracic air sac is very large, it occupies the largest
part of the cavum subpulmonale, and the posterior thoracic air sac is a very
small structure (Figs. 6 a, 10 a, 13). In penguins the anterior thoracic sac is very
small. In all song birds also it is extremely small, but always recognizable
as narrow space directly behind the lung hilus. Yet in these species it has a larger
opening into the interclavicular air sac, thus fusing with the latter (Fig. 15).

The posterior thoracic air sac is divided in two sacs on each side of the
body in storks only. Well developed laterobronchi pass into each of the two
air sacs directly at the margin of the lung. It can be concluded from their con-
nexion to two laterobronchi, lying directly beside each other, that these two
sacs, the middle and posterior thoracic air sacs, are corresponding to the posterior
thoracic air sac of all other birds. The anterior thoracic sac which originates
always close to the hilus from the third ventrobronchus, and has its second
ostium at the lung margin, in storks as well as in all other species, is unambigu-
ously marked by these connexions. Therefore this newly added air sac of storks
cannot be derived from the anterior thoracic air sac.

The thoracic air sacs always significantly differ from the cervical and interclavicular sacs in that way that never any kind of structures or tissue bridges
pass through their open space (Figs. 7 a, b, 11, 13, 15, 16 a–c, 17 a–e). Also, diver-

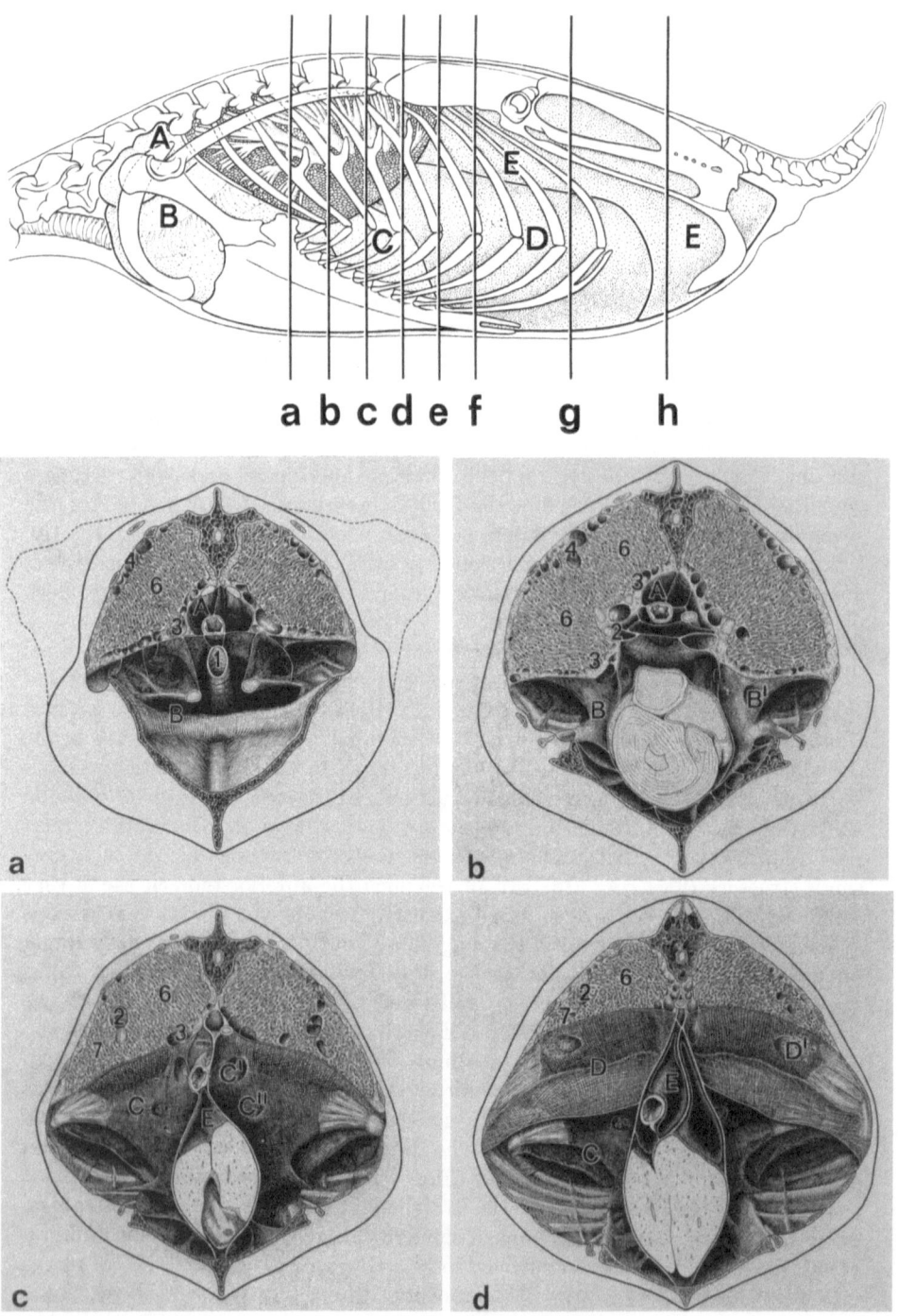

Fig. 16a–d. (Legend see p. 57)

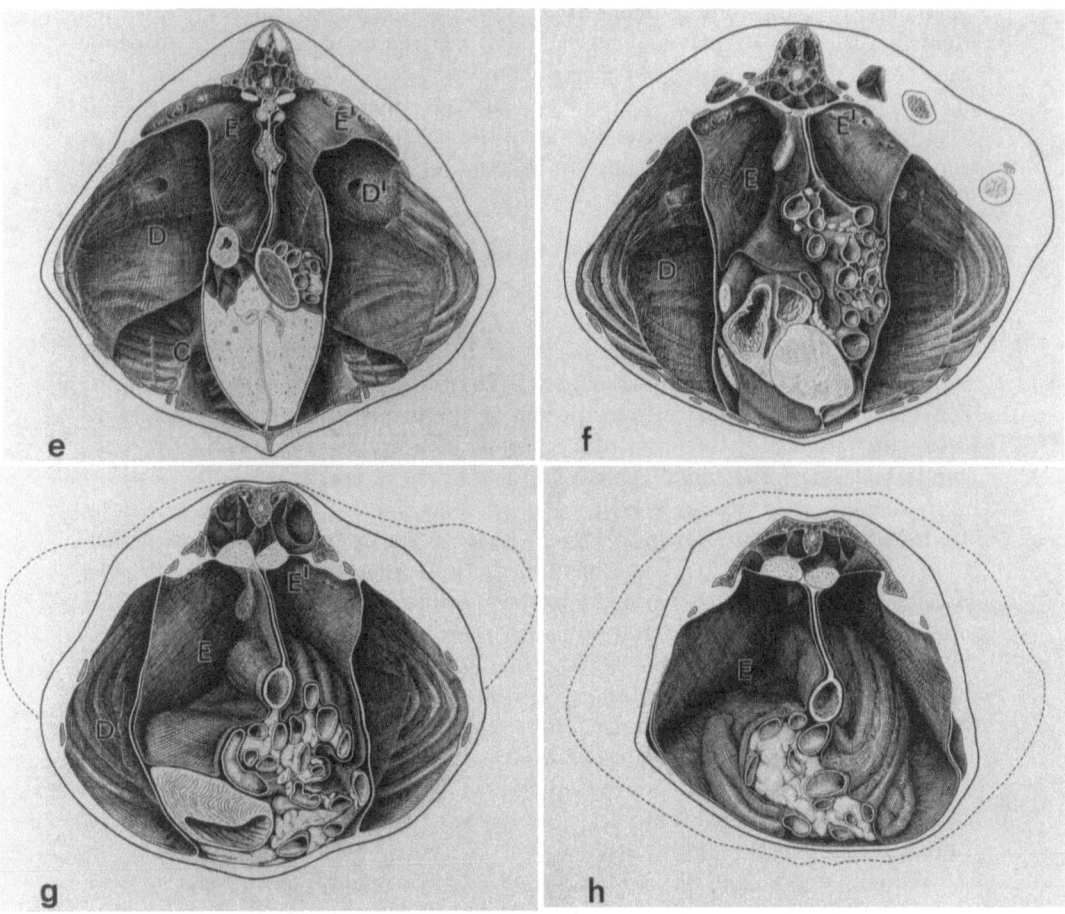

Fig. 16e–h

Fig. 16a–h. Mute swan, *Cygnus olor*, series of cross sections of the trunk. At a lateral view of the trunk the positions of the sections in their relations to lungs, air sacs and skeleton have been marked. The cross sections are always viewed from caudal. a) Section through the anterior lung and the anterior end of the sternum, esophagus, trachea and Aa. carotides are cut. In the continuation of the horizontal septum, a medial separating wall between the cervical (A) and the interclavicular (B) air sacs can be seen. Pneumatic spaces in vertebrae, ribs, sternum and other trunk bones, as will be seen in the following cross sections also. b) Section through the middle of the lung and the heart, the atria and ventricles of which have been cut. The great cardiac vascular stems and the bifurcation of the trachea are visible. c) Section through the lung shortly behind its middle with its primary bronchus and through the anterior liver between the two oblique septa. The heart tip is still visible, above the liver the esophagus is situated, still above that the aorta. Laterally, in the horizontal septum the Mm. costopulmonales are exhibited, medially the main ostia (C') of the cut anterior thoracic air sac (C). d) Section through the posterior lung with primary bronchus and large ostium (D') into the posterior thoracic air sac (D) which is cut in the dorsal cavum sub-pulmonale, underneath the anterior thoracic air sac (C). Between the oblique septa the liver and esophagus, dorsally the cranial part of the abdominal air sac (E). e) Section directly caudal to the lung with the dorsal ostia (E') into the abdominal air sac (E) which expands dorsal to the viscera in the cavum cardioabdominale. Laterally, between the oblique septa ticula into the surrounding organs are only seldom originating from them. Individual, larger air sac diverticula can be found between esophagus and pericardium and between esophagus and liver, especially in species gulping large boli. These diverticula generally originate from the anterior thoracic air sac, more seldom also from the posterior thoracic sac, as in the cormorant. Small diverticula into the sideways adjacent sternal ribs can be found originating also from the anterior thoracic air sac.

III. The Abdominal Air Sac

While the air sacs discussed above all lie ventral to the lungs, separated from the lung only by the horizontal septum and from the visceral cavity by the oblique septum, the abdominal air sacs are situated behind the lung and behind the oblique septum in the region of the intestinal tract. They are paired and completely similar constructed. They originate from the end of the primary bronchus, which penetrates that portion of the horizontal septum which ascends towards dorsal at the caudal margin of the lung. The ostium lies in the lateral part of the posterior margin and opens into a relatively large sac (Figs. 7b, 11, 13, 15, 16e–h, 17f–h). In its lateral portion the single large ostium of the primary bronchus, similar to the ostium of the laterobronchus into the posterior thoracic air sac, in most species receives openings out of the lateral parabronchial net of the lung. These openings, when present in a large number, may be joined together into a saccobronchus, as in numerous duck species (Fig. 25a), or they may completely replace the main ostium, as in song birds (Figs. 25c, 26c). These openings of a lateral parabronchial lung net condensed into a secondary ostium or a saccobronchus, are completely lacking in penguins and emus; they are present in all other species, to a very varying degree, however (Figs. 23–26). Starting at the primary and secondary ostia, which always lie close to each other, the sac expands into a funnel at first and then into a balloon.

With its dorsal wall the abdominal air sac completely grows together with the dorsal abdominal cavity wall, extending from lateral as far as to the median mesentery covering the kidneys and adrenal glands. Gonads and their efferent

and body wall the posterior thoracic air sacs (D), ventrally the anterior thoracic air sacs (C) still cut. In the mesentery, dorsally the ovary and adrenal glands, ventral to the synsacrum the head of the kidneys. f) Section above the hip joint. Larger abdominal air sacs (E) dorsally in the abdominal cavity, ventrally the tip of the liver, gizzard and intestinal convolutions. Lateral to the oblique septa the posterior thoracic air sacs (D). Large pneumatic spaces in the synsacrum. g) Section caudal to the hip joint through the most caudal part of the posterior thoracic air sacs (D) above the attachment of the oblique septa to the lateral body wall. Large abdominal air sacs (E) on both sides of the mesentery and dorsal to the intestinal bulk. Dorsal to the kidneys large pneumatic spaces in the pelvis. h) Section caudal to the oblique septa and the posterior thoracic air sacs. The abdominal air sacs (E) fill the largest part of the abdominal cavity. Ventrally the visceral bulk, dorsal to the kidneys the pneumatic spaces.—A cervical air sac with ostium A', B interclavicular air sac with ostium B', C anterior thoracic air sac with ostium C', D posterior thoracic air sac with ostium D', E abdominal air sac with ostium E'. 2 primary bronchus, 3 ventrobronchi, 4 dorsobronchi, 5 laterobronchi, 6 parabronchi between dorsobronchi and ventrobronchi, 7 additional parabronchial net between primary bronchus and posterior air sacs pathes are not covered, however. Caudally the fusion of air sac wall and kidney has variable extensions, at least it reaches as far as the middle of the abdominal cavity, often even the rectum (Figs. 13, 15). More or less distant from the root of the mesenteries, passing straight through the sac, the air sac wall becomes free and descends into the abdominal cavity (Figs. 11, 13, 15, 16d–h, 17f–h).

Cranially and laterally the wall of the abdominal air sac has spread around its ostium and widely upon the oblique septum, growing together with the latter (Figs. 11, 12, 14, 16d–h, 17f–h). The fusion extends along the lateral wall of the abdominal cavity as far as its middle level, caudally often far beyond the extension of the oblique septum. The abdominal air sac lies in the abdominal cavity like a balloon grown together dorsally and laterally, the rest of the wall portions of which are freely mobile against the viscera (Figs. 11, 12, 14, 16d–h, 17f–h).

In penguins and rheas, the walls of the abdominal air sac are considerably coarse and short so that both opposite sacs, even if maximally filled, do not displace the whole visceral tract. In these species, the dorsal and lateral fusions of the air sac walls are more limited (Fig. 11). In all other birds the abdominal air sac is significantly larger and wider and possesses a wide spread field of fusion. Moreover its wall has been developed to such an extent (Figs. 12, 14), that the sac filled maximally with air on one side alone is able to occupy more than the total abdominal cavity. The walls are so thin that they cannot be prepared without being partially destroyed. This extremely wide and delicate air sac wall is always found to a smaller or greater degree strangulated between the individual intestinal loops, indeed even compressed. Generally the enormous extension of the walls still allows enough variation of mobility for the various filling phases of the abdominal air sacs. In individual species I observed openings into the abdominal cavity in the dorsal region. However, it is not clear as yet whether the whole abdominal cavity has become an air sac functionally, in the living animal already, or whether these findings are postmortal changes.

The two abdominal air sacs from dorsal and lateral enclose the mesentery and the bulk of intestinal convolutions (Figs. 16d–h, 17f–h). Their extension is limited in penguins, rheas and loons, in all other species they reach as far as the cranial part of the abdominal cavity and caudally, the cloaca (Figs. 16a–h, 17f–h). There the abdominal air sacs may fuse ventrally to the rectum and widely communicate with each other. Because of their thin walls they give a negative form of the viscera (Figs. 9, 10a, b). At the same time the air sacs have the possibility of varying their volume and the viscera may occupy various filling phases without a change in the external body form.

Dorsally the abdominal air sacs extend in the form of diverticula, namely lateral to the kidneys, within their field of fusion. From there they penetrate into the pelvis, between kidneys and pelvis, around the hip joint and partly even into the femur. The extent of this pneumatisation varies, corresponding to other parts of the body, in relation to the systematic position, the way of life and size. In some mute swans I observed a communication through the posterior oblique septum between posterior thoracic and abdominal air sac.

No structures or tissue bridges pass through the abdominal as well as the thoracic air sacs. Contrary to all other air sacs the abdominal sac is not separated from the viscera by a septum and therefore not stretched. Its size is always

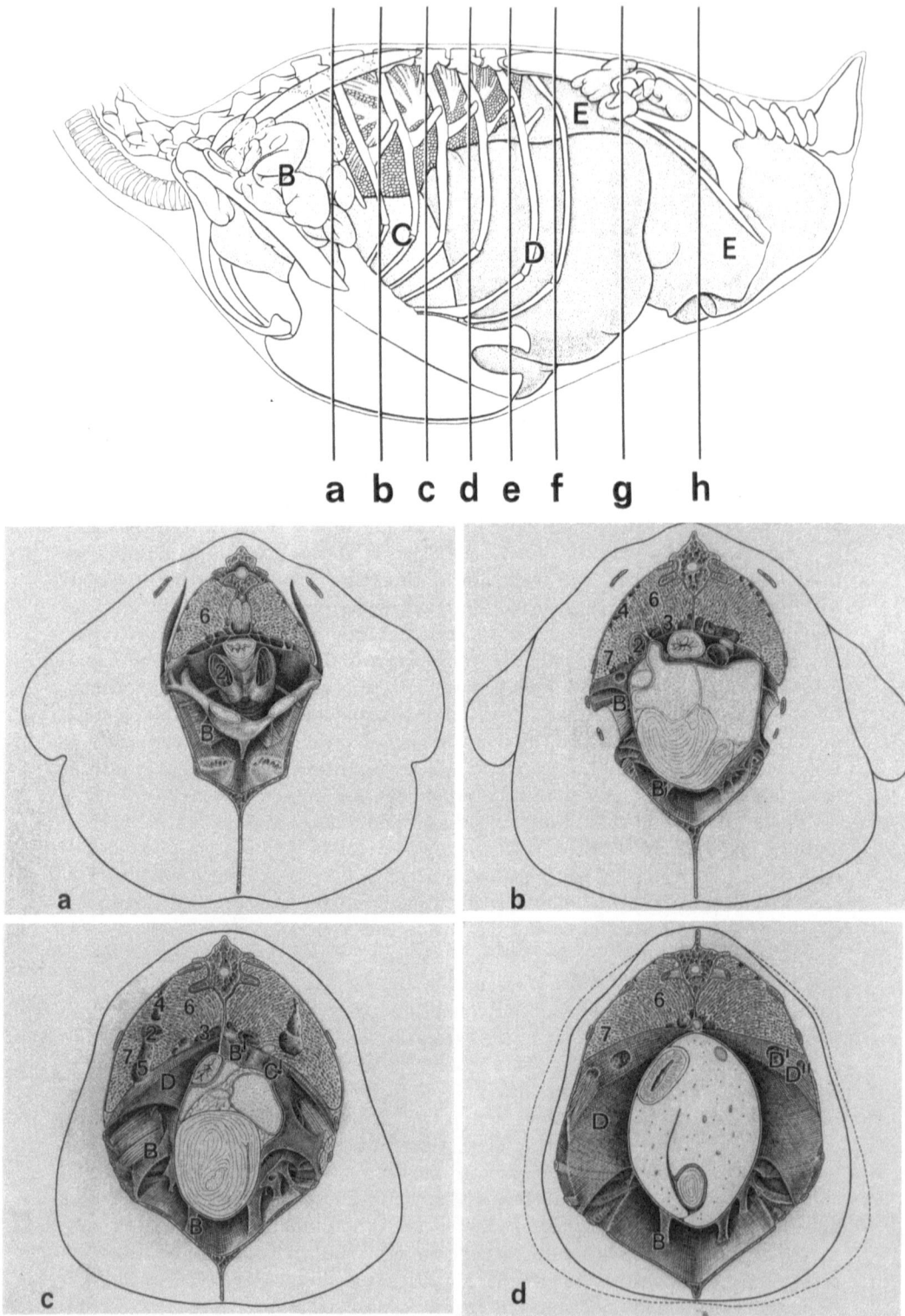

Fig. 17 a–d. (Legend see p. 61)

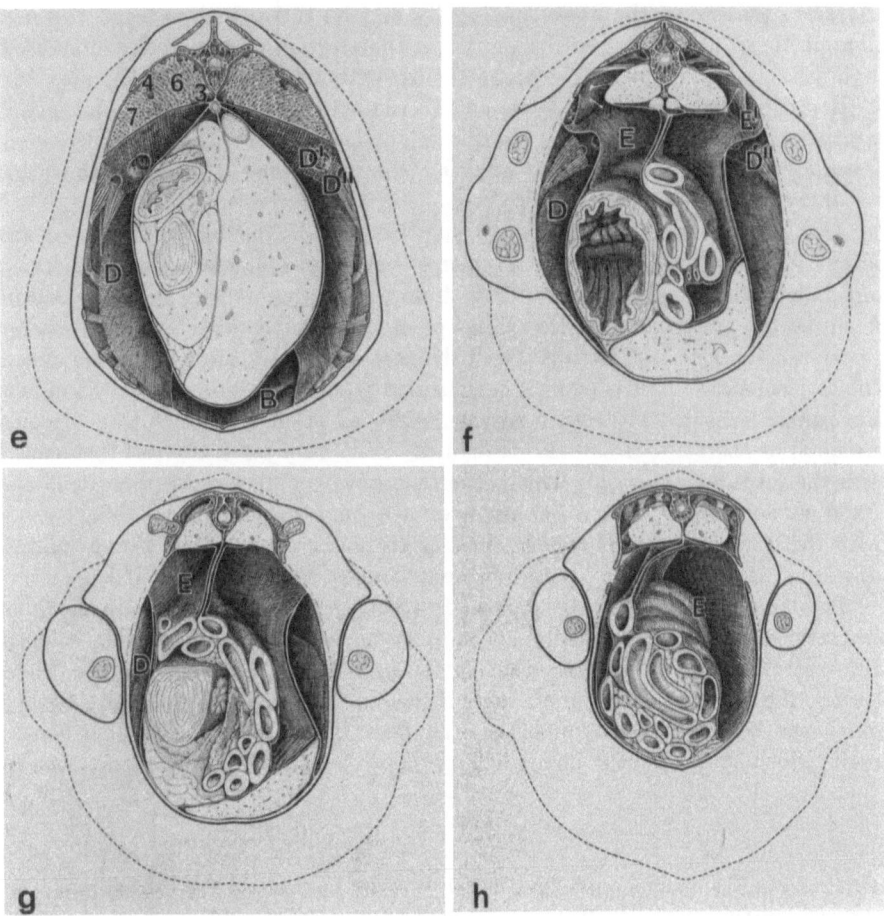

Fig. 17 e–h

Fig. 17 a–h. Carrion crow, *Corvus corone*, series of cross sections through the trunk. At a lateral view of the trunk the positions of the sections in their relation to lungs, air sacs and skeleton have been marked. The cross sections are always viewed from caudal. a) Section through the anterior lung and the anterior end of the sternum. Esophagus, primary bronchi behind the bifurcation of the trachea and Aa. subclaviae at the anterior margin of the pericardium are cut in the interclavicular air sac (*B*). Besides the pneumatisation of the vertebrae, ribs, the sternum and other trunk bones as in all following sections, also a diverticulum of the interclavicular air sac between thoracic wall and scapula is cut. b) Section through the anterior lung and the anterior heart with atria and orifices of the ventricles. Between heart and lungs the esophagus and the primary bronchi just at the entrance into the lung hilus are situated. Ventral to the heart the impar median diverticulum of the interclavicular sac (*B*). c) Section through the middle of the lung at the origin of the large laterobronchus (5) and through the middle of the heart which together with the esophagus is surrounded by the pericard/oblique septum transition. The ostium into the interclavicular (*B'*) and into the anterior thoracic air sac (*C'*) are seen, medial and lateral to the lung hilus. These two air sacs are fused in song birds. d) Section through the posterior lung and the heart tip. In the horizontal septum lies the ostium (*D'*) out of the laterobronchus and (*D''*) out of the accessory parabronchial net (7) between primary bronchus and posterior air sacs into the cut posterior thoracic air sac (*D*). The horizontal septum contains the Mm. costopulmonales related to the size of the abdominal cavity and its filling with viscera. The left abdominal sac, at the side of the gizzard, is therefore generally more compressed than the opposite (Figs. 10a, 16d–h, 17f–h), without having a smaller size due to its construction. Small birds are able to reduce the volume of the abdominal cavity in such a manner, that the abdominal air sacs are almost totally compressed, while large birds as swans may compress their abdominal sac also, yet always maintain a large residual volume of air.

As a normal value, nine air sacs may be stated. The cervical air sacs are paired, the interclavicular air sac is impar, the anterior thoracic, posterior thoracic and abdominal air sacs are all paired. A larger number of sacs was only found in storks the posterior thoracic air sac of which is subdivided in a medial and a posterior thoracic sac. Reductions of the normal number are found more often. The cervical air sac pair is lacking in loons and grebes. In all other species studied this pair is present, yet often relatively small, as in song birds. In these species the anterior thoracic air sac also is reduced, often very markedly and then fused with the interclavicular sac. This is the reason why only five large air sacs are found in song birds. All other air sacs are only diverticula which originate from the large air sacs. However, directly from the dorsomedial margin of the lung small diverticula may pass into neighbouring vertebrae and ribs.

The large air sacs may be divided in two groups. The first group includes the cervical and interclavicular air sacs, to which in song birds also belongs the ventral part of the latter reaching far in a caudal direction, and in these species, the anterior thoracic air sacs. Numerous structures like vessels, nerves and tissue bridges pass through these air sacs. They lie in that region of the trunk which only slightly changes its volume during respiratory movements.

at its margin. The oblique septa have united ventrally and enclose the visceral bulk with liver and proventriculus. The oblique septa are attached to the sternum via fibrous tissue bridges. e) Section through the posterior lung. View into the large posterior thoracic air sac with its two ostia (D') and (D''). The oblique septa are closed around the bulk of gizzard and liver, ventral to this bulk of viscera lies the impar median diverticulum of the interclavicular air sac (B). f) Section caudal to the lung and the sternal end, above the hip joint. The oblique septa have attached behind the end of the sternum to the ventrolateral body wall. Between them lies the bulk of viscera, with liver, gizzard and intestinal convolutions, dorsally the abdominal air sacs (E). Above these, kidneys and adrenal glands and the pneumatic spaces between pelvis and kidneys can be seen, as in the two following sections also. g) Section through the hip joint and the caudal part of the posterior thoracic air sacs before the attachment of the oblique septa to the lateral body wall. Between the oblique septa lies ventrally the visceral bulk with gizzard, liver and intestinal convolutions, dorsally the abdominal air sacs (E) expand below the kidneys. h) Section through the trunk caudal to the posterior thoracic air sacs. The abdominal cavity is filled by the intestinal convolutions and the two abdominal air sacs (E) which extend on both sides of the mesentery, dorsally beneath the pelvis lie the kidneys and the pneumatic spaces.—A cervical air sac, B interclavicular air sac with ostium B' and the ostium C' of the anterior thoracic air sac which has fused with the interclavicular, D posterior thoracic air sac with the laterobronchial ostium D' and the ostium out of the accessory parabronchial net D''. E abdominal air sac. 2 primary bronchus, 3 ventrobronchi, 4 dorsobronchi, 5 laterobronchi, 6 parabronchi between dorsobronchi and ventrobronchi, 7 accessory parabronchial net between primary bronchus and posterior air sacs

The second group is formed by the two pairs of the posterior thoracic and the abdominal air sacs to which, according to development and position, the pair of the anterior thoracic air sacs may be added. These air sacs are always large and have smooth walls, have no structures passing through and lie in that portion of the trunk which can very well be dilated and compressed.

Topography and Branchings of the Bronchial System

The bronchial system of the avian lung may not be compared with the bronchial tree of the mammalian lung, since it does not have dichotomous, dendritic, blindly ending branchings of the bronchi. The primary bronchus, partly bipennately, gives off three groups of a limited number of secondary bronchi, without substantially changing its character (Figs. 18, 30 a–c, 31 b, 32 a–c, 33 a–c, 34 a–c). Directly at the lung hilus the four, in storks five (Fig. 32 b), ventrobronchi originate, extending on the ventral surface of the lung. A portion of the primary bronchus, free of branchings, follows. The primary bronchus after it has bent towards caudal, gives off two to five laterobronchi towards ventral (Figs. 24 a–c, 26 a–c, 30 a, b, 32 a–c, 33 a–c). On the other side of the primary bronchus, in its middle to posterior part, seven to ten dorsobronchi originate (Figs. 18, 24 a–c, 26 a–c, 30 a, b, 32 a–c, 33 a–c). The dorsobronchi branch on the dorsolateral side of the lung. From the whole surface of all secondary bronchi, directed towards the lung, the parabronchi originate, which run parallelly and cross link. They connect the two layers of the secondary bronchi to each other (Figs. 18, 27 a, b, 30 a–c, 31). Thus no blind endings are existent in the bronchial system of birds, all pathes into the bronchial system lead back to the primary bronchus (Figs. 18, 31). In the mantle of the parabronchi the network of blood and air capillaries has been developed. There the gas exchange takes place.

The air sacs are connected to the bronchial system in a very characteristic manner. The cervical air sacs always originate from the first ventrobronchus more or less far distant from the lung tip (Figs. 20 c, 28 a, b, 29 a–c). The interclavicular and the anterior thoracic air sacs always originate near the lung hilus, from the third ventrobronchus near its branching from the primary bronchus (Figs. 20 c, 21 c, 22 c, 28 a, b, 29 a–c). Moreover, these air sacs at the lateral lung margin beside the hilus have a connection into the parabronchial net originating from lateral branches of the first to third ventrobronchi (Figs. 21 c, 22 c, 28 a, b, 29 a–c). The posterior thoracic air sac is always connected to the primary bronchus by a wide laterobronchus and the abdominal air sac receives the entering primary bronchus which has a wide lumen (Figs. 18, 24 a–c, 26 a–c, 28 a, b, 29 a–c). These simple connections for the posterior air sacs are only found in penguins, emus, cormorants and storks.

In the storks already, a connection between the two posterior air sacs and the primary bronchus and the laterobronchus, respectively, is developed by interposition of a parabronchial net. In storks and cormorants this network is existent only to a very limited extent (Figs. 23 a, 24 a, 32 b), in herons and ducks, in plovers, curlews and sandpipers, it is already well developed (Figs. 23 b, c, 24 b, c, 25 a, 26 a, 32 c, 33 a) and reaches its highest differentiation in fowllike and song birds (Figs. 25 b, c, 26 b, c, 33 b, c). In these species is the abdominal

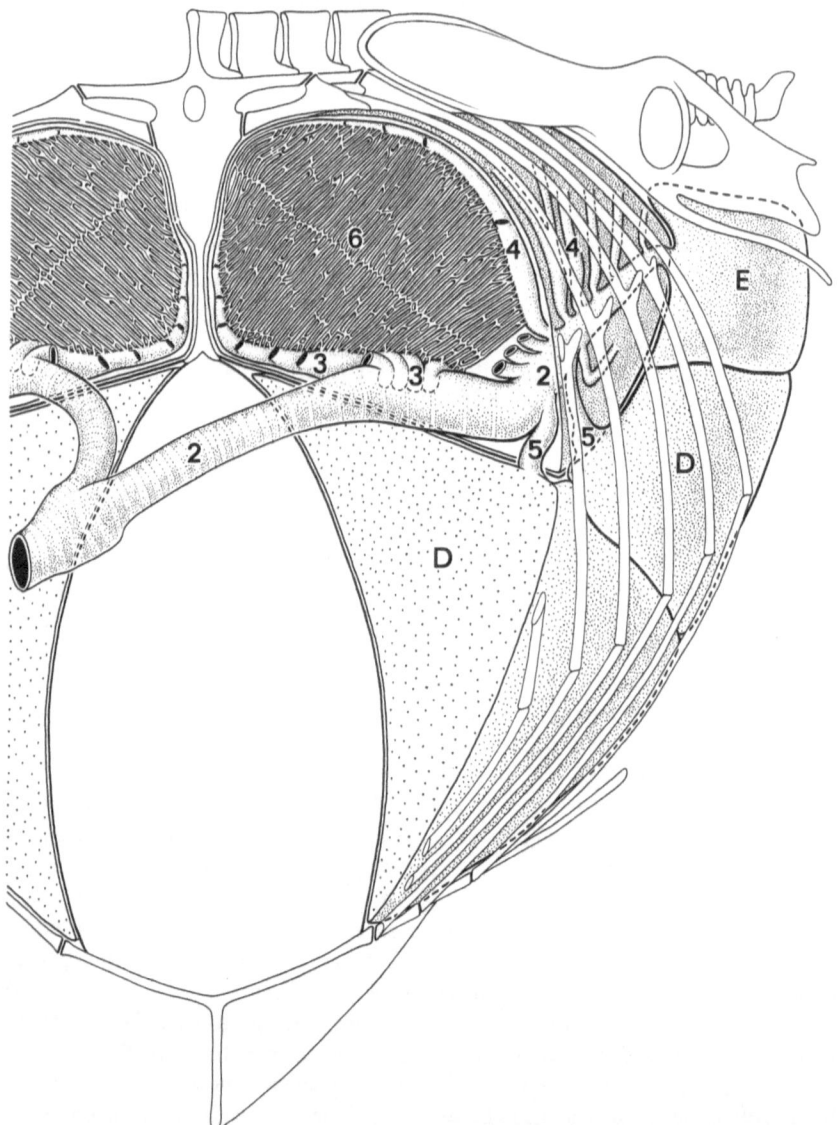

Fig. 18. Idealized cross section through an avian body, basing on a lung air sac preparation of a white stork, *Ciconia ciconia*. View from cranial on the posterior part of the preparation, out of which only the primary bronchus (2) projects. The lungs lie above the horizontal septum, beneath them, between body wall and oblique septa the air sacs are developed. The primary bronchus (2) enters the lung from ventromedial and gives off the group of ventrobronchi (3). After it has reached the lung surface, the group of dorsobronchi (4) originates. Between them and the ventrobronchi the parabronchi (6) are situated connecting these secondary bronchi as a three dimensional network. The primary bronchus (2) continues into the abdominal air sac (E). Opposite to the dorsobronchi the laterobronchi (5) originate, which through their wide lumen communicate with the posterior thoracic air sacs (D). (All other families of birds have only one posterior thoracic air sac and thus only one large laterobronchus connecting it)

air sac connected functionally to the primary bronchus only via parabronchi. The parabronchi, often gathered into larger bronchi, open as saccobronchi into the posterior air sacs (Figs. 23 c, 24 c, 25 a–c, 26 a–c).

I. The Primary Bronchus

The trachea enters the thoracic cavity at its ventromedian part and passes through the interclavicular air sac (Figs. 13, 15, 16 a, b, 17 a, b, 27 a, b). Very shortly after its entrance or not until immediately before the lung hilus occurs the division into the primary bronchi at the bifurcation, generally accompanied by the formation of an often very complicatedly structured syrinx. In ducks the large resonance bullae are situated at the trachea and the primary bronchus in the region of the bifurcation (Fig. 19 a, b). In penguins the trachea is doubled starting already at the upper neck, in the bifurcation the two primary bronchi separate without a marked formation of a syrinx.

The primary bronchus then passes obliquely from ventral, medial and cranial through the horizontal septum into the lung, about in the middle of the line of its greatest thickness (Fig. 18). It forms the lung hilus together with the A. pulmonalis, entering cranial and a little lateral to the primary bronchus, and the V. pulmonalis issuing caudal and a little medial to it (Figs. 13, 15, 19 b, 20 c, 21 c, 22 c, 28 a, b, 29 a–c). The primary bronchus maintains its direction from medioventral to dorsolateral and thus passes through the medial lung until it touches the lateral lung surface, where it appears a little caudal to the middle of the lung and just above its inferior margin. At this point the primary bronchus turns towards caudal and runs parallely and just above the inferior margin of the lung in a posterior direction, to open into the abdominal air sac at the caudal lung margin (Figs. 18, 20 a, 23 a, 24 a). This course of the primary bronchus is the same in all avian lungs. Without additional structures and therefore very easy to observe, is the course of the primary bronchus in penguins and emus, cormorants and storks.

While the primary bronchus enters the lung obliquely from anterior, ventral and medial, it begins to give off four or five ventrobronchi on its dorsal side (Figs. 18, 30 b, 31, 32 a–c, 33 a–c). The opening into the first ventrobronchus is shifted a little towards lateral while the following openings are always a little more medially. During the ramification of the ventrobronchi, the cross section of the primary bronchus increases about 25%. Without any further changes in diameter it passes up to the lateral lung surface. Along this portion the primary bronchus does not give off any branches (Figs. 18, 30 b, 31, 32 a–c, 33 a–c).

Angulation, width of openings and increase of the diameter of the ventrobronchi after their origin from the primary bronchus, and increase of the cross sectional area of the primary bronchus in the course of the ventrobronchial branching, can be found in a correspondent manner in all species studied. The lungs of different species, however, show enormous differences in size and thickness (Figs. 20 b, 21 b, 22 b). Consequently, the portion of the primary bronchus free of branchings (measured from just behind the last ventrobronchial branching to the lung surface) is of very different length. In penguins, loons and grebes with flat lungs (Fig. 32 a) this portion is short; it is longer, however, in species

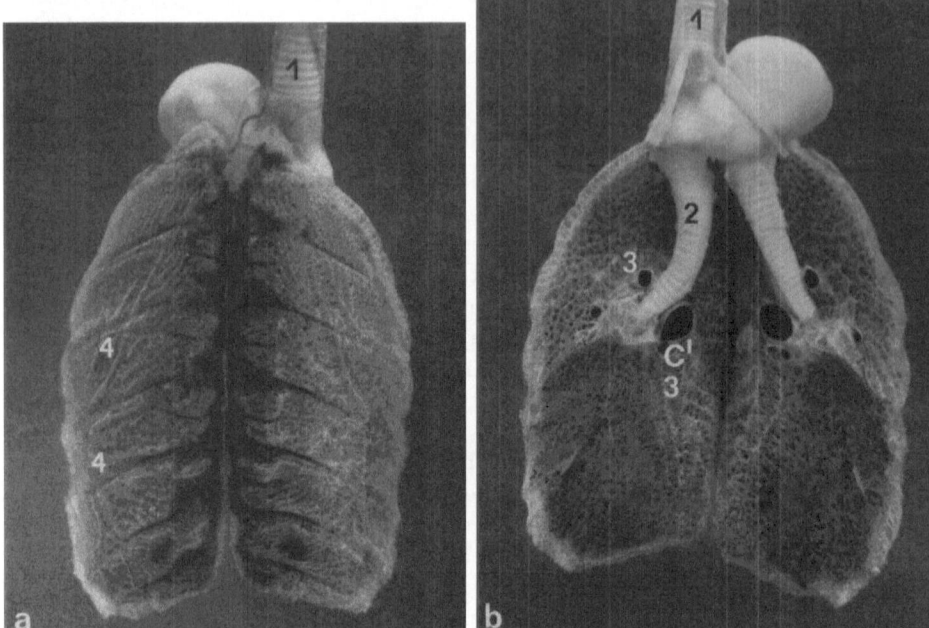

Fig. 19a and b. Fixed lung preparation of a northern mallard, *Anas platyrhynchos*, a) seen from dorsal, b) from ventral, ×0.9. Cranially the lungs have a tip and caudally they end with a transverse line. Incisures of the ribs visible on the dorsal surface, then the superficially passing dorsobronchi (*4*). On the ventral side the trachea (*1*) with the bifurcation in the two primary bronchi can be seen. At the bifurcation is the bulla which is so typical for many male duck species. Cranial to the primary bronchus the A. pulmonalis enters the lung hilus, caudal to it the V. pulmonalis exits. Besides, there the ostia into the interclavicular and anterior thoracic (*C'*) air sac are situated. Single branches of the ventrobronchi (*3*) can be seen

with thick lungs, as for instance swans and storks (Fig. 32b, c). If the portion, free of branchings, is short, the primary bronchus is relatively wider and vice versa. In species with very short primary bronchi, the curve of the bronchus towards caudal is pushed into the portion of free branchings. Thus a vestibulum is formed (Fig. 32c), while in species with thicker lungs and longer primary bronchi a straight tube, bent at its end, is formed (Fig. 33b). It is conformable to the literature, to always use the term "vestibulum" for that portion of the primary bronchus that is devoid of branchings.

Starting at the point where the primary bronchus reaches the lateral lung surface and bends in a caudal direction, it begins to give off dorsally the series of the dorsobronchi (Figs. 18, 20a, 23a, 24a, 32a, b). In penguins and cormorants the first dorsobronchus originates on the cranial side of the primary bronchus that is flattened a little at the lung surface; in a dorsal direction the next dorsobronchi follow (Figs. 20a, 23a, 24a, 32a, b). The intervals between their origins are continually increasing for the posterior dorsobronchi, at the same time the originating dorsobronchi become increasingly smaller (Figs. 18, 20a, 23a, 24a,

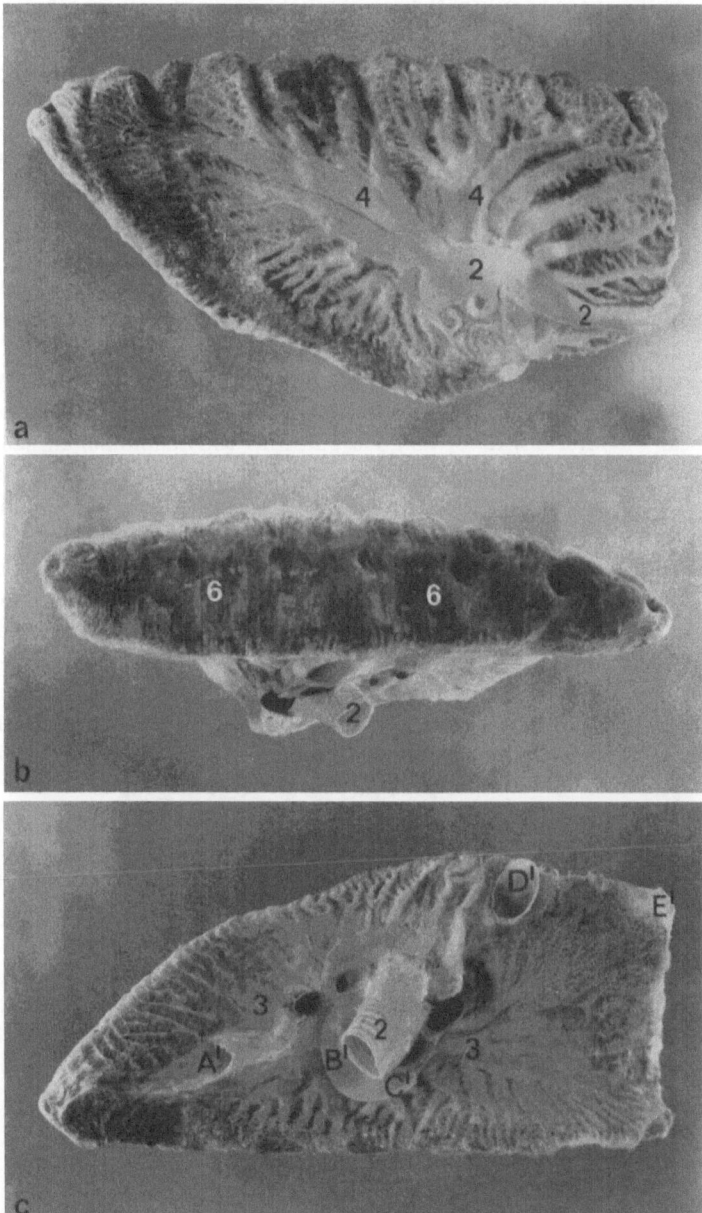

Fig. 20a–c. Fixed preparation of the left lung of a king penguin, *Aptenodytes patagonica*, a) from dorsolateral, b) from medial, c) from ventral. ×0.5. On the dorsolateral surface the primary bronchus (*2*) and the group of dorsobronchi (*4*) can be recognized. The medial side shows the deep incisures of the ribs and the parabronchial net (*6*) between dorsobronchi and ventrobronchi, additionally the lung hilus directed towards ventral. The ventral side exhibits the entering primary bronchus (*2*) and the ventrobronchi (*3*), besides the ostia into the cervical (*A'*), interclavicular (*B'*) and anterior thoracic (*C'*) air sacs as well as the ostia into the posterior thoracic (*D'*) and abdominal (*E'*) air sac

32 a, b). At the opposite side of the dorsobronchi, the primary bronchus gives off on its ventral side the small group of the laterobronchi. Since the primary bronchus, after it touches the lateral side of the lung surface, turns in a slight dorsal curve towards caudal, the dorsobronchi stand on the convexity of this curve, the latero-bronchi in the concavity and thus directly opposite to the medial dorsobronchi (Figs. 18, 20 a, 23 a, 24 a, 32 a, b). On the inside of the primary bronchus the originating laterobronchi connect with the first dorsobronchi via crestlike pro-cesses across the wall of the primary bronchus, in a few species, as in penguins for instance.

While the primary bronchus gives off dorsobronchi towards the dorsal side and laterobronchi towards the ventral side, it becomes narrower proportionately to the number of branching secondary bronchi. After the last secondary bronchus has originated, the primary bronchus still possesses about 20% of the vestibular cross section. As relatively well marked primary bronchus it then passes, parallel to and near the lateral inferior lung margin, into the abdominal air sac, entering at the caudal lung margin with a funnel-shaped dilatation (Figs. 18, 20 a, 24 a, 32 a, b). These relations may be observed directly on the lateral lung surface of penguins and emus, storks and cormorants.

But in all other avian families too, the primary bronchus may be found in this form: oblique entrance into the lung hilus from ventromedial and crowded branching of four ventrobronchi, forming an acute angle towards craniodorsal and spreading on the ventral surface of the lung. By the dilatation of the primary bronchus, the more or less distinct vestibulum is formed along the following, obliquely passing stretch. This is especially marked for a short interval between beginning of the vestibulum and lung surface, for a thickset primary bronchus, as in song birds. The primary bronchus then turns caudally and starts to give off 7 to 10 dorsobronchi, which fan out on to the dorsolateral surface of the lung (Figs. 24 a–c, 26 a–c, 30 a, b, 31, 32 a–c, 33 a–c). The origin of dorso-bronchi extends along the further course of the primary bronchus as far as shortly before its entrance into the abdominal air sac. Ventrally, opposite to the medial dorsobronchi, originate the 2–5 laterobronchi. In the course of the origination of the dorsobronchi and laterobronchi the primary bronchus con-tinually becomes narrower in all species, proportionately to the number of branching secondary bronchi, to open into the abdominal air sac with a cross sectional area reduced to 20% or even less (Figs. 24 a–c, 26 a–c, 30 a, b, 31, 32 a–c, 33 a–c).

This structure of the primary bronchus is in most avian families subject to change only in so far, as also parabronchi originate from the primary bronchus behind the vestibulum, besides the dorsobronchi and laterobronchi. They always originate from the ventral and lateral side of the primary bronchus. The para-bronchi form a network stretched out in the direction of the primary bronchus and pass towards the abdominal and posterior thoracic air sacs, where they open into the lateral part of the funnel-shaped dilatations of the primary and laterobronchus. A few of them only are present in storks and cormorants (Fig. 32 b). In cranes, ducks, swans, plovers, curlews, sandpipers and auks the number of parabronchi originating from the primary bronchus increases, they form a com-pact bulk with their network which extends corresponding to its origin lateral

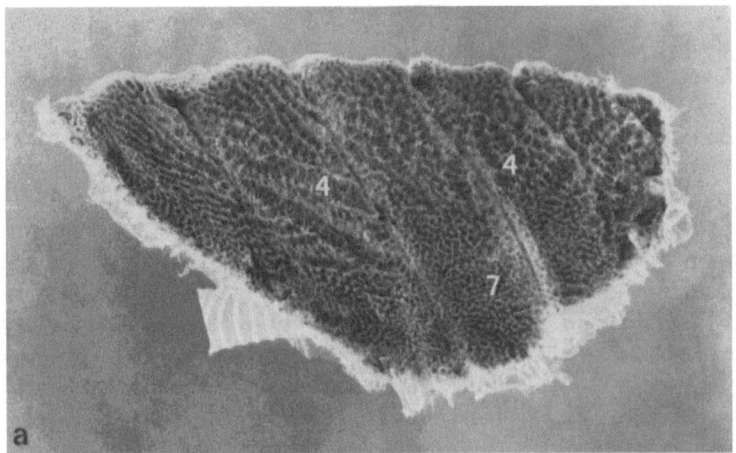

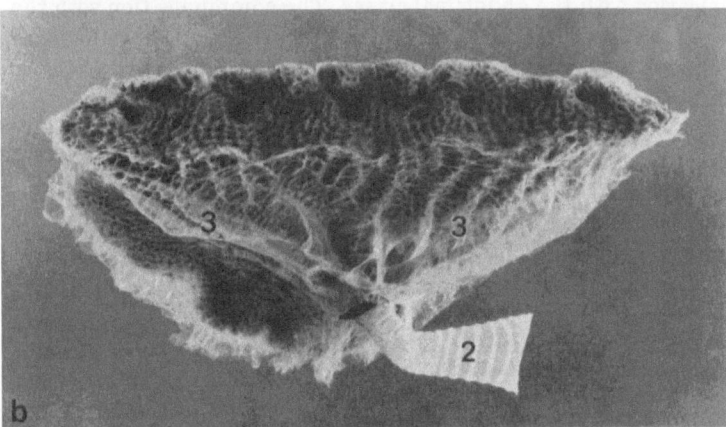

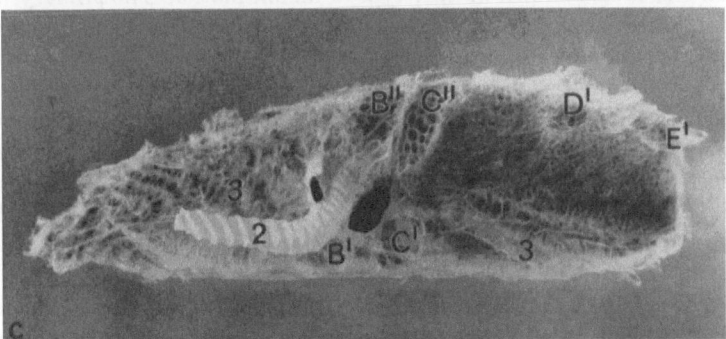

Fig. 21 a–c. Fixed preparation of the left lung of the grey heron, *Ardea cinerea*, a) from dorso-lateral, b) from medial, c) from ventral, ×1.0. On the dorsolateral surface the extremely thin walled dorsobronchi (*4*), in their initial portion covered by the parabronchial network (*7*) between primary bronchus and posterior air sacs. The medial surface shows the deep incisures caused by the ribs and the extremely high and thin walled ventrobronchi (*3*). The primary bronchus (*2*) enters the lung at its deepest point. From ventral the A. pulmonalis is shown cranial to the primary bronchus, caudal to it the V. pulmonalis. Medial to the lung hilus the primary ostia (*B'*) (*C'*), lateral to the hilus the secondary ostia into the interclavicular (*B''*) and anterior thoracic (*C''*) air sac, caudally at the lung margin the ostia into the posterior thoracic (*D'*) and abdominal (*E'*) air sac. Openings into the parabronchi shine through the thin walled ventrobronchi (*3*)

and ventral to the primary bronchus (Figs. 21a, 23b, c, 24b, c, 25a, 26a, 31, 32c, 33a). Thereby, the primary bronchus is shifted from the lung surface and the inferior margin, respectively, so far into the depth of the lung that it is displaced towards medial and a little dorsal. On the surface of the lung the primary bronchus cannot be seen anymore, instead a network of parabronchi (Figs. 21a, 23b, c, 25a).

If the number of parabronchi, which originate from the posterior part of the primary bronchus, increases again, the primary bronchus is not only shifted but also narrowed towards the caudal lung margin. Thus it becomes increasingly thinner in swans, fowllike birds, pigeons and gulls (Figs. 26b, 30a, b, 31, 32c, 33a, b, 34b, c). In the song birds, the primary bronchus has become so narrow after branching of the last dorsobronchus that it cannot be distinguished from a parabronchus (Figs. 26c, 33c). Here the parabronchial net alone mediates the communication with the abdominal air sac. The communication with the posterior thoracic air sac is also taken over, to a large part at least, by this parabronchial net, however a well developed laterobronchus always remains as connection between primary bronchus and this air sac (Figs. 24b, c, 26a–c, 30a, b, 31, 32b, c, 33a–c, 34b, c). Accompanying the more marked extension of the parabronchial net, originating from the primary bronchus, parabronchi also originate from the external sides of the initial portions of dorsobronchi, so that the dorsobronchi too are shifted towards deeper portions of the lung. This starts in ducks and swans (Figs. 25a, 26a, 31, 32c), continues in gulls and pigeons and is most marked in fowllike and song birds (Figs. 25b, c, 26b, c, 33b, c).

II. The Secondary Bronchi

The difference between the avian bronchial system and the mammalian bronchial tree is also shown in their type of denomination. The primary bronchus completely passes the whole lung. The secondary bronchi branch in groups as large bronchi from the primary bronchus. The majority of them pass at the lung surface, for once dorsolaterally and second ventrally (Figs. 18–22, 30a–c, 31, 32a–c, 33a–c, 34a–c). According to their position within the individual groups the secondary bronchi branch at the plane of the surface, at first manyfold. This generally happens in an unipennate or bipennate manner, all lateral ramifications passing at the lung surface. Their branches, lying beside each other, consequently supply more or less wide regions. The term secondary bronchus includes its main trunk with all its ramifications, independent of its size, the degree of ramification and the number of branches. Towards the inside of the lung the secondary bronchi at their total surface give off a large number of parabronchi, and with their terminal branches also terminate into parabronchi.

The Ventrobronchi

The first four secondary bronchi, which originate from the primary bronchus directly at its oblique entrance into the lung hilus and spread at the ventral side of the lung, are ventrobronchi. Their initial openings are situated on the dorsal side of the primary bronchus, arranged in an oblique line (Figs. 30b, 31,

32a–c, 33a–c). The first ventrobronchus originates a little laterally on the dorsal side of the primary bronchus, the following a little further medially each, so that their openings lie on an axis passing directly craniocaudally and intersecting the primary bronchus that runs obliquely from ventromedial to dorsolateral in an acute angle. These initial openings are oval, oriented transverse to the longitudinal axis of the primary bronchus, and have a diameter about $^3/_4$ the size of the diameter of the primary bronchus at the lung hilus. The longitudinal axes of these oval openings are normally oriented transverse to the longitudinal axis of the primary bronchus, a fact that is partly caused by their crowded sequential arrangement. Thus these openings are separated from each other only by very narrow lips which are only of the same thickness as the extremely thin ventrobronchial wall. These lips, too, end directly at the level of the wall of the primary bronchus.

In their first portion, directly adjoining the origin, all ventrobronchi pass in a cranial direction. Their axis forms an angle towards cranial with the axis of the obliquely passing primary bronchus, which very constantly amounts to about 45° in the different species (Figs. 31, 32a–c, 33a–c). After this short initial portion the ventrobronchi very markedly dilate, often as much as a manyfold of the diameter of their initial opening (Figs. 28a, b, 29a–c). This is possible, because the ventrobronchi, in their further course, part from each other and pass in various directions. Yet with all their branches they always lie directly at the ventral surface of the lung (Figs. 28a, b, 29a–c).

The first ventrobronchus runs straight towards cranial. Shortly after its origin it has the same size as the primary bronchus, in a few species, for instance in herons (Fig. 21b) it may even by far exceed the diameter size of the primary bronchus. After a short unbranched portion, it gives off a well developed lateral branch, which itself gives rise to small ramifications for the lateral lung margin, and in its course turns so far caudally around the A. pulmonalis that the artery is almost completely enclosed by the first ventrobronchus and its lateral branch (Figs. 28a, b, 29c). While this behaviour is met in most birds, in penguins, loons, swans and song birds, the first branch of the first ventrobronchus may also pass in a laterocaudal direction caudal to the A. pulmonalis, as in the white stork. This branch of the first ventrobronchus passes parallel to the lateral lung margin beyond the hilus in a caudal direction. Thus it supplies the inferior lung surface lateral to the hilus. The main stem of the first ventrobronchus, passing on towards cranial, then ramifies into a number of branches which pass towards the medial and lateral lung margin. A better developed main branch is directed towards the cranial lung tip and sends off smaller branches towards both margins (Figs. 32a–c, 33a–c). More or less distant from the lung tip a second, mostly short yet well developed branch leaves the main branch, which shortly afterwards opens into the ostium of the cervical air sac (Figs. 20c, 28a, b, 29a–c).

The second ventrobronchus regularly is very small. After a short course towards cranial it splits up, T-like in two branches, one of which is running towards the medial lung margin, supplying a variously broad section of the ventral lung surface, medial to the lung hilus, adjoining the region of supply of the first ventrobronchus (Figs. 31, 32a–c, 33a–c). The second branch turns towards lateral and a little caudal. Generally it passes through the furca of the

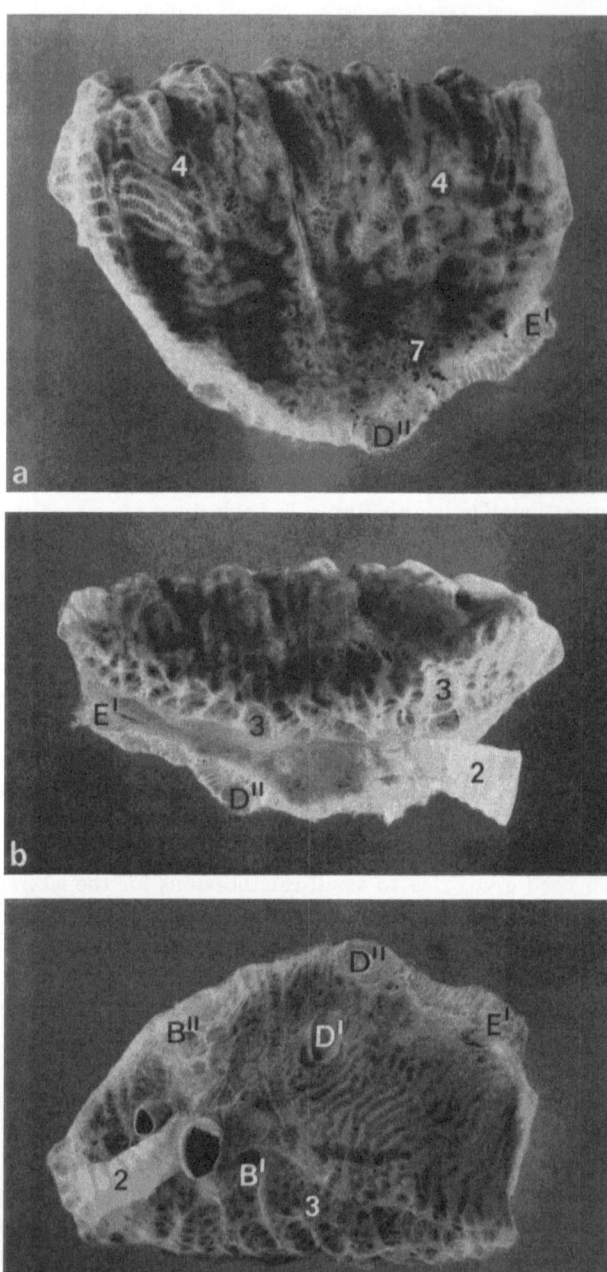

Fig. 22a–c. Fixed preparation of the left lung of a black-throated jay, *Garrulus glandarius*. a) from dorsolateral, b) from medial, c) from ventral. ×2.5. On the dorsolateral side only the terminal branches of the dorsobronchi (*4*) can be recognized, the network of parabronchi (*7*) between primary bronchus and posterior air sacs occupies the posteroinferior part of the surface. On the medial side the thin walled ventrobronchi are exhibited besides the deep incisures of the ribs. The ventral side shows the pulmonary artery before and the pulmonary vein behind the primary bronchus (*2*), the thin walled ventrobronchi (*3*), and the ostia into the interclavicular (*B′*) (*B″*), posterior thoracic (*D′*) and abdominal (*E′*) air sac

A. pulmonalis, which is formed by one branch running towards cranial and the other branch running towards caudal. This lateral branch of the second ventrobronchus from medial joins the branch of the first ventrobronchus, that runs in a caudal direction, in supplying the region lateral to the lung hilus. The second bronchus too, similar to all others, after its first course, directed cranially experiences a marked dilatation of its cross section. The first and second ventrobronchi regularly supply the cranial half of the inferior surface of the lung in all birds.

Lateral to the lung hilus, the first branch of the first ventrobronchus and the branch of the second ventrobronchus running laterally give off a series of very short, usually vesicle-shaped branches together with their terminal branchings. These short branches, as all other ventrobronchi, give off parabronchi into the interior of the lung. Besides, they are connected to the interclavicular and the anterior thoracic air sac through the horizontal septum and thus form the variously wide additional ostia for these two air sacs. In a few species only, as in storks and rheas, these two branches of the first and second ventrobronchus, or one of them, continue as a larger bronchus with a funnel-shaped dilatation directly into these ostia (Figs. 11, 32 b). In most birds the communication between air sacs and ventrobronchi consists only of the system of larger, vesicular dilatations, connected to each other.

The third ventrobronchus regularly is much larger than the second, however not quite as large as the first. After a short course towards cranial, it turns in a caudal direction and runs towards caudal, medial to the primary bronchus, near the medial lung margin. It supplies the caudal half of the ventral surface of the lung. The lateral section of this surface, which contains the large ostia into the posterior air sacs, remains devoid of ventrobronchial supply (Figs. 28 a, b, 29 a–c, 32 a–c, 33 a–c). The third ventrobronchus gives off branches for the medial lung margin and caudally gives rise to a few lateral branches, too. The third ventrobronchus is characterized by a short, sturdy stem, which it gives off towards medioventral shortly after its origin from the primary bronchus. This bronchial stem penetrates the horizontal septum and is divided in the ostium for the interclavicular air sac, directed cranially, and the ostium for the anterior thoracic air sac, directed caudally (Figs. 11, 13, 15, 28 a, b, 29 a–c). Also in song birds, in which interclavicular and anterior thoracic air sacs have fused, this stem is divided in two ostia which open into the fused air sacs (Figs. 15, 29 c). In storks, the third ventrobronchus is divided in two ventrobronchi which between them divide the area of supply. The first of these two (the third in our counting) forms the ostium into the interclavicular air sac, the following (the fourth) the ostium into the anterior thoracic air sac.

The fourth ventrobronchus (in storks the fifth) immediately follows the third on its lateral side as a much weaker secondary bronchus (Figs. 28 a, b, 29 a–c, 32 a–c, 33 a–c). It has only a few ramifications, sometimes they may be completely lacking. If the fourth ventrobronchus is better developed, and if the lung of a larger animal is studied, it often gives off a sturdy branch which, caudal to the lung hilus, runs transversely towards lateral, as in the rhea, in swans (Fig. 32 c), grey heron and in many other species. If the fourth ventrobronchus is poorly developed, the third ventrobronchus may give rise to this branch transverse

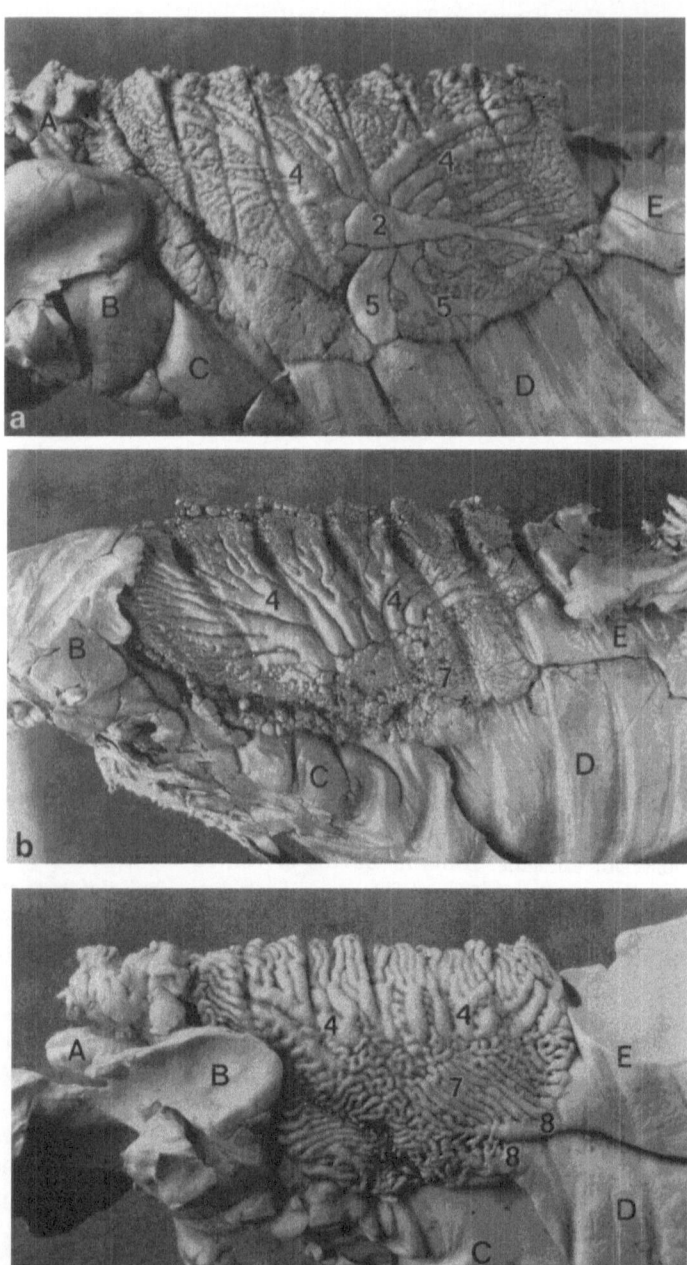

Fig. 23a–c. Lung-air sac preparations from dorsolateral, left side. a) Green cormorant, *Phala-crocorax aristotelis*, ×0.9. The primary bronchus (*2*) reaches the lateral surface, gives off the dorsobronchi (*4*) and laterobronchi (*5*) and bends towards caudal into the abdominal air sac. b) Crowned crane, *Balearica pavonina*, ×0.6. Only the dorsobronchi (*4*) are visible at the surface. Primary and laterobronchi are covered by the parabronchial network (*7*) between primary bronchus and posterior air sacs. c) Golden plover, *Pluvialis apricaria*, ×1.3. Besides the dorsobronchi (*4*) the well developed saccobronchi (*8*) and the parabronchial network (*7*), extended from them to the posterior air sacs can be seen. — *A* cervical, *B* interclavicular, *C* anterior and *D* posterior thoracic air sac, *E* abdominal air sac

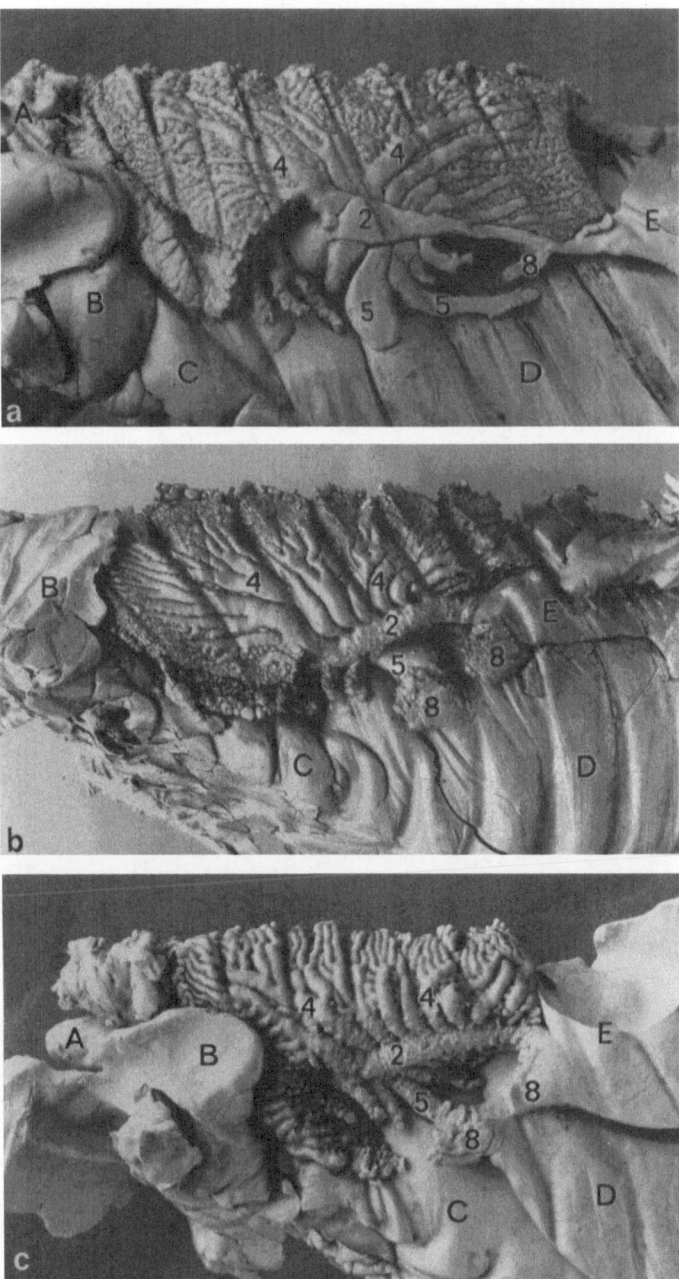

Fig. 24a–c. Lung air sac preparation of Fig. 23, posterior primary bronchus (*2*) prepared and its air sac connections demonstrated. a) Green cormorant, ×0.9. Only a small saccobronchus (*8*) present at the posterior primary bronchus (*2*). Connection of the posterior thoracic air sac (*D*) without saccobronchi. b) Crowned crane, ×0.6. Solid, short saccobronchi (*8*) for the abdominal (*E*) and posterior thoracic (*D*) air sac. c) Golden plover, ×1.8. Highly developed saccobronchi (*8*) for the posterior air sacs. — *5* laterobronchi, *A* cervical, *B* interclavicular, *C* anterior thoracic, *D* posterior thoracic, *E* abdominal air sac

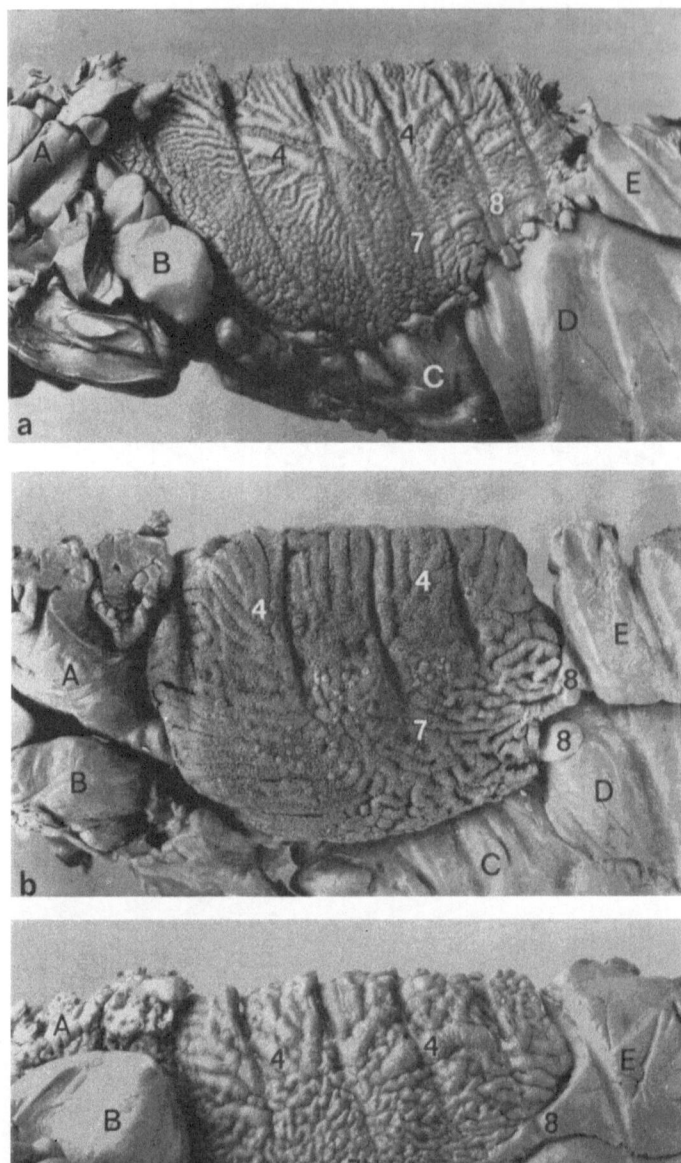

Fig. 25a–c. Lung air sac preparations from dorsolateral, left side. a) Northern mallard, *Anas platyrhynchos*, ×0.9. At the lung surface only the superior portions of the dorsobronchi (*4*) and the long saccobronchus (*8*) into the abdominal air sac can be seen, the caudal part of the surface is occupied by the parabronchial net (*7*) between primary bronchus and posterior air sacs. b) Domestic fowl, *Gallus domesticus*, ×1.1. All bronchi reaching the surface have respiratory tissue in their walls, the atria of which may be seen in their contours. Saccobronchi (*8*) into the posterior air sacs. c) Carrion crow, *Corvus corone*, ×1.5. Upper portions of the dorsobronchi (*4*) and saccobronchi (*8*) into the posterior air sacs visible, highly developed parabronchial net into the posterior air sacs. — *A* cervical, *B* interclavicular, *C* anterior thoracic, *D* posterior thoracic, *E* abdominal air sac

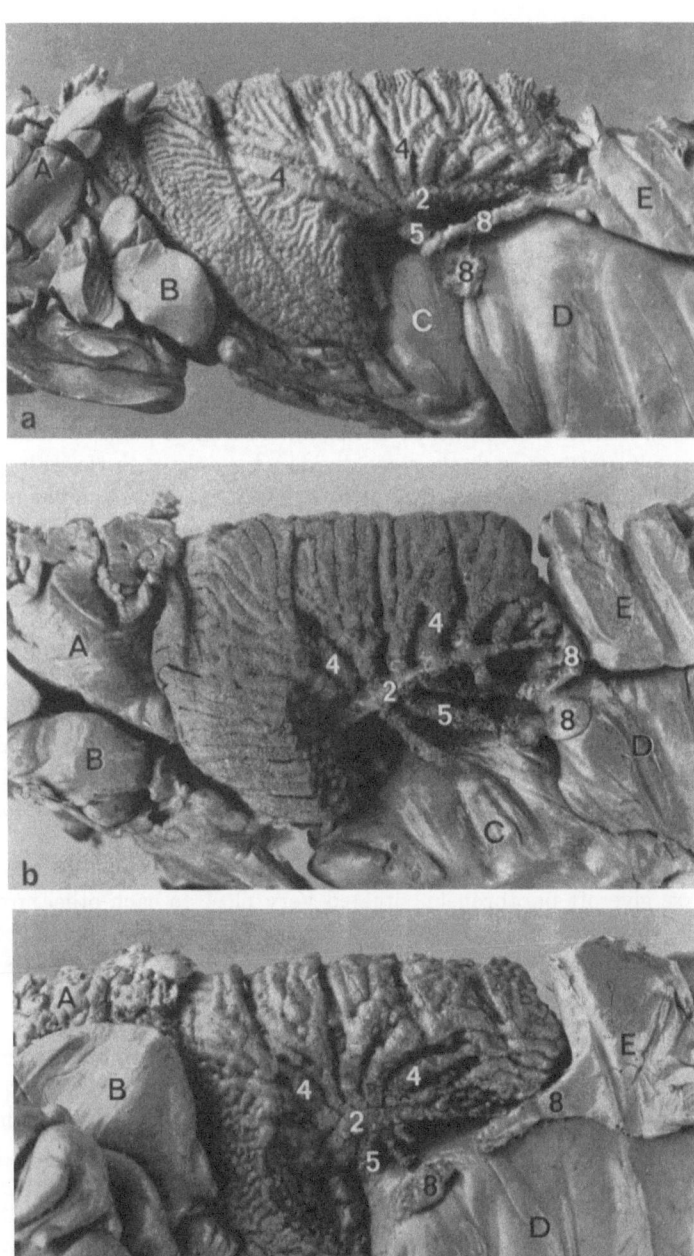

Fig. 26a–c. Lung air sac preparation of Fig. 25, posterior primary bronchus (*2*) prepared with air sac connections. a) Northern mallard, ×0.9. Very long saccobronchus (*8*) into the abdominal air sac (*E*), a short one into the posterior thoracic air sac (*D*). b) Domestic fowl, ×1.1. Primary bronchus becomes very narrow towards the abdominal air sac (*E*), instead, a large saccobronchus (*8*) as connection, similar to the connection of the posterior thoracic air sac. c) Carrion crow, ×1.5. Primary bronchus (*2*) into the abdominal air sac (*E*) becomes narrower than a parabronchus. Large saccobronchi. — *A* cervical, *B* interclavicular, *C* anterior, *D* posterior thoracic, *E* abdominal air sac

to the lateral lung side, as in grebes. In the narrowly constructed lung of penguins this branch is completely lacking. The anterior branch of the pulmonal vein issues, medial to the primary bronchus, between first and second ventrobronchus, the medial branch of the V. pulmonalis between second and third ventrobronchus, and the posterior branch of the V. pulmonalis between fourth ventrobronchus and its lateral branch. This is also true for storks if the division of the third ventrobronchus is considered.

The ventrobronchi come to lie close to each other directly, wall to wall, with their main stems and all branches, at the ventral surface of the lung. Rarely, any deviations from this rule may be found, as in storks, in which small amounts of adipose tissue lie between the ventrobronchial stems. Not each of these closely crowded main and lateral branches of the ventrobronchi possesses a lateral wall of its own, but often enough they are divided by only a single wall. On their ventral side the ventrobronchial wall is formed by an uninterrupted membrane which gives rise to septa that subdivide the ventrobronchi in main and lateral branches. Not until the margins of the ventral lung surface the numerous ramifications separate into individual branches. Still they remain arranged in a single layer beside each other and thus all together pass around the medial margin of the ventral surface, a little distance on to the medial surface of the lung towards dorsal (Fig. 27 a, b). Not until there they split up in parabronchi. In the same way, the united branches of the two first ventrobronchi run around the cranial and lateral margin of the ventral surface on to the dorsolateral surface of the lung, namely caudally as far as the deepest lateral point of the lung (Fig. 23 a, c). There they pass a various distance obliquely towards dorsal and caudal, before they ramify as parabronchi.

The ventrobronchi do not only end as parabronchi, but also along their whole course give off parabronchi, situated very close to each other, from their dorsal side which are directed towards the interior of the lung. These parabronchi pass obliquely or perpendicularly into the interior lung (Figs. 18, 31, 32 a–c, 33 a–c). Only the initial portions of the main stems are devoid of parabronchi, because the great lung vessels are situated on these portions and don't leave room for parabronchi (Figs. 31, 32 a–c, 33 a–c). Therefore the ventrobronchi are perforated along their wall directed towards the interior of the lung, by the openings into the parabronchi. It is a remarkable fact that the openings into the parabronchi become smaller the nearer they are situated to the primary bronchus and the larger is the size of the ventrobronchus. However, this is developed to its fullest extent only in penguins. The parabronchi themselves, except in penguins, only very sligthly or not at all increase in diameter anywhere between primary bronchus and lung margin. If the ventrobronchial opening into the parabronchi is very narrow, the parabronchi recover to their normal diameter directly behind this opening.

Not considering the relations discussed above, the ventrobronchi as a system display a significant variety of their width. In storks they are thin and therefore do not connect each other with their branches in all parts of the ventral surface of the lung, but partly let their parabronchial net lie close to the surface, and, besides, are only developed as flat tubes. In most other birds they are closely connected to each other and by this form a closed layer at the ventral side of

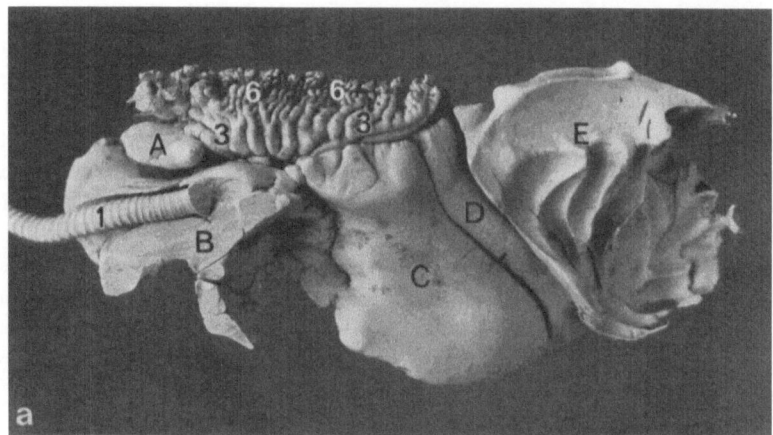

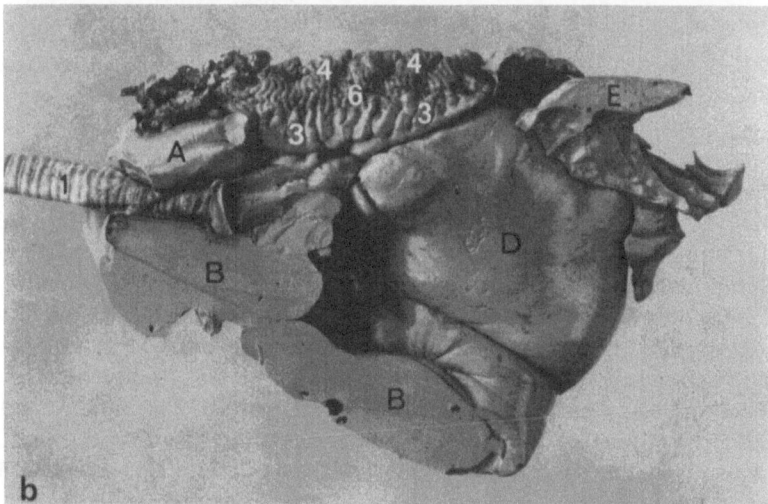

Fig. 27a and b. Half of a lung air sac preparation, from medial. a) Golden plover, *Pluvialis apricaria*, ×1.1. All air sacs can be seen, impar interclavicular air sac (*B*) cut in the median line. Anterior (*C*) and posterior (*D*) thoracic air sacs smoothly limited by the oblique septum against the abdominal cavity, abdominal air sac (*E*) with impressions of the viscera. Lung with terminal branches of the ventrobronchi (*3*) and connected parabronchi (*6*) on the medial side. b) Carrion crow, *Corvus corone*, ×0.9. Interclavicular air sac, medially cut, with large medioventral diverticulum. Abdominal air sac (*E*) only partly filled. Medial surface of the lung with incisures of the ribs; from ventral the ventrobronchi (*3*) reach the medial surface. Above of it parabronchi (*6*) between dorsobronchi (*4*) and ventrobronchi (*3*). *1* Trachea, *A* cervical air sac

the lung, their branches having about the same height and width. In the grey heron on the other hand the ventrobronchi have about a height double as great as their width (Fig. 21 b), thus making up a large part of the lung thickness. Less marked is the ventrobronchial height in a number of song birds as thrushes, jays and crows (Fig. 22 b).

A more profound variety is only existent for the width of the ventrobronchi. Origin and angle of ramification, arrangement and course are quite constant in all birds. From the first ventrobronchus, if present, always the cervical air sacs originate, from the third ventrobronchus stem the openings into the interclavicular and anterior thoracic air sacs. The additional ostia for these two air sacs, lateral to the lung hilus, stem from the terminal ramifications of the caudal branch of the first and the lateral branch of the second ventrobronchus. On their side directed towards the anterior of the lung the ventrobronchi give off parabronchi, and with their terminal ramifications also form a parabronchial net, these two types of parabronchial origin continually overlapping each other. It is remarkable that in some species the initial openings of the parabronchi are small near the primary bronchus and become increasingly larger towards the periphery, the ventrobronchi on the other hand decreasing in size.

The Dorsobronchi

Behind the vestibulum of the primary bronchus, the seven to ten secondary bronchi originate dorsally, which as dorsobronchi spread towards the lateral and dorsal lung surface. This is independent of the fact, whether the primary bronchus touches the lateral lung surface, as in penguins, emus, cormorants and storks, or whether it passes beneath the lateral surface in the interior of the lung, as in all other birds (Figs. 24a–c, 26a–c, 30a, b, 32a–c, 33a–c). In the portion of the arc of the primary bronchus running towards caudal the first dorsobronchi originate. The first dorsobronchus has its transversely oval opening on this arc directly on its cranial side. Sometimes, however, it is shifted a little towards dorsal. The dorsobronchi, which directly follow to the first opening, having transversely oval to round openings, originate already on the dorsal side of the primary bronchus that runs towards caudal. The more caudally the dorsobronchi originate, the greater become the intervals between their round initial openings. Thus the primary bronchus on its dorsal side is occupied by the originating dorsobronchi as far as shortly before its caudal end where it opens into the abdominal air sac. The dorsobronchi originate not only with increasing intervals between each other — from cranial to caudal — but their initial openings also become increasingly smaller towards caudal, correlating to the decreasing width of the primary bronchus. Therefore the size of the dorsobronchi also decreases continually from cranial to caudal (Figs. 24a–c, 26a–c, 30a, b, 32a–c, 33a–c).

The round to transversely oval openings of the first dorsobronchi occupy the total dorsal width of the primary bronchus. The round openings of the middle and caudal dorsobronchi which are farther apart become increasingly smaller, however. They have a smaller diameter than the primary bronchus at their origin. The cranial and middle dorsobronchi are directed strictly towards cranial in their initial course, forming an angle of about 45° with the longitudinal axis of the primary bronchus. Only the two or three last dorsobronchi are bent towards caudal beginning at their origin. As soon as the first dorsobronchi fan out and take their position at the plane of the lung surface, they dilate, while the following dorsobronchi dilate in their wall directed towards cranial, immediately after

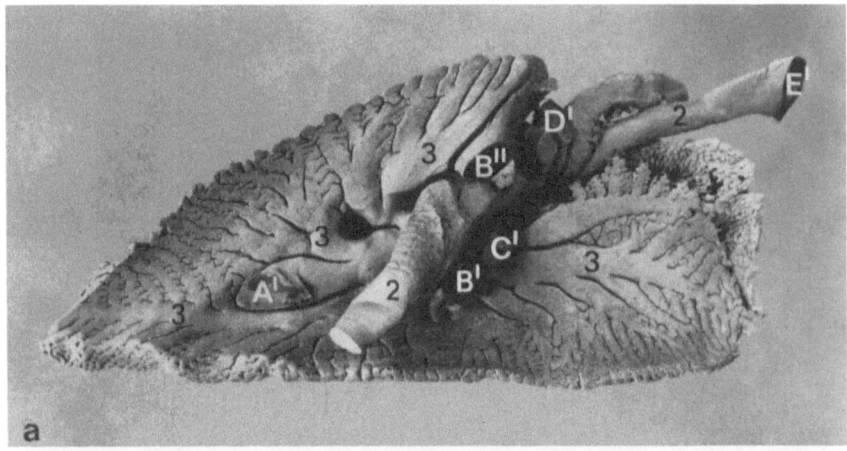

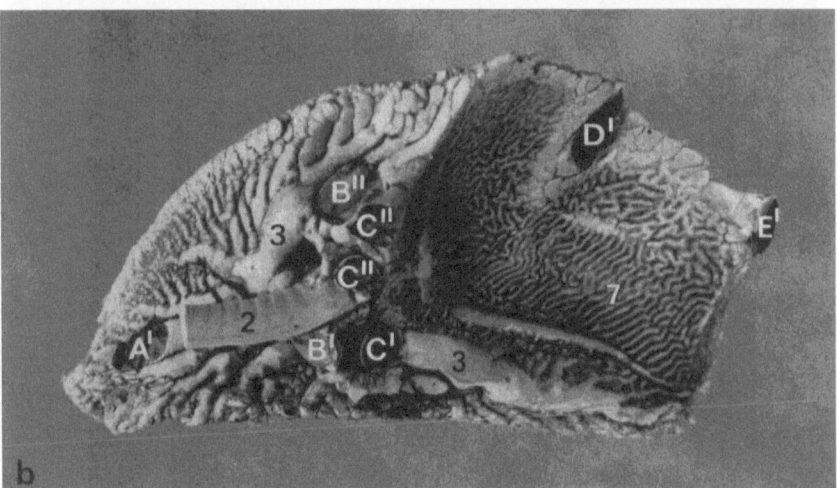

Fig. 28a and b. Different lung forms and various positions of the air sac ostia. The ventrobronchi occupy the surface. Lung injection preparations from ventral. a) King penguin,
Aptenodytes patagonica, ×0.5. Ostia into the cervical (A'), interclavicular (B') and anterior
thoracic (C') air sacs originating from the ventrobronchi, posterior thoracic air sac (D')
from a short laterobronchus, abdominal air sac (E') from the primary bronchus, and accessory
ostium into the interclavicular sac (B''). b) European pochard, *Aythya ferina,* ×1.5. Besides
ostia of the ventrobronchi into the anterior air sacs, accessory ostia into the interclavicular
(B'') and anterior thoracic (C'') air sac lateral to the lung hilus. On the caudal lung surface
network of parabronchi (7) between primary bronchus and posterior sacs. — *2* primary bronchus,
A' ostium for the cervical, B' for the interclavicular, C' for the anterior, D' for the posterior
thoracic air sac and E' ostium for the abdominal air sac

their penetration through the relatively narrower initial opening in the wall of
the primary bronchus. Thus the direction of the initial bronchial course towards
cranial is manifested. This dilatation is very marked in penguins, similarly in
the cormorants (Figs. 23a, 24a, 32a). In most other species this dilatation si
not as marked, extending along a longer portion of the dorsobronchus (Figs. 23b,

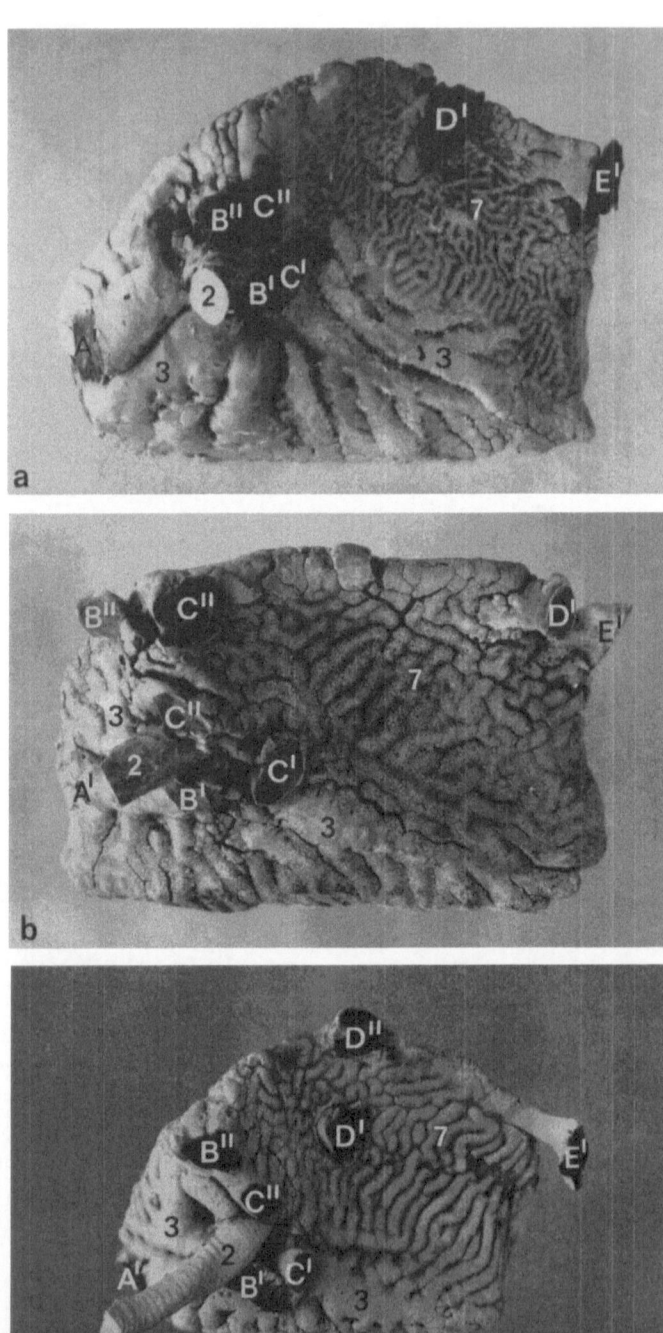

Fig. 29a–c. Different lung forms and positions of the air sac ostia. Lung injection preparation
from ventral. The ventrobronchi occupy the surface above the lung hilus, caudally beside
them the parabronchial net (7) between primary bronchus and posterior air sacs. a) Black-

24 b, 25 a, 26 a, 30 a, 32 c), so that the dorsobronchi gradually show a significantly larger cross section than at their origin, as in song birds (Figs. 25 c, 26 c, 33 c).

Regularly the first dorsobronchus is the largest, except in the penguin where the second is even larger. All following become smaller towards caudal. The first bronchus runs towards dorsocranial, the following arrange themselves in a fan-like manner, the middle bronchi running towards dorsal and the posterior turning increasingly towards caudal. The first dorsobronchus gives off its crowded and continually branching ramifications in an unipennate form only towards cranial and ventral. In very wide lungs, as in ducks and swans, the first dorsobronchus gives rise to well developed branches perpendicularly towards ventral, shortly after its origin from the primary bronchus. These branches supply the most ventral part of the triangular lung from its lateral surface (Figs. 26 a, 30 a, 32 c). The next dorsobronchi bifurcate more like a furca, especially towards dorsal; the second gives off its branches towards craniodorsal, this is especially marked in penguins, where the third branch shows the same behavior. Corresponding to their own course, the middle and posterior dorsobronchi give off their branches mostly towards dorsal and caudal (Figs. 24 a–c, 26 a–c, 32 a–c, 33 a–c). The dorso-bronchi integrate in a plane in the dorsolateral lung surface by a close apposition of their branches. They show a behaviour similar to the ventrobronchi. However, the neighbouring walls never fuse to such an extent with each other that their superficial wall runs across a number of dorsobronchi, as is true for the greater, proximal portion of the ventrobronchi.

The dorsobronchial fan reaches the dorsal margin of the lung, where it possesses its last ramifications before the transition into parabronchi, in the course of the curvature on to the medial lung surface. Since the ventrobronchi run around the anterior lateral margin of the lung, in a zone varying from species to species, on to the dorsolateral side of the lung, the dorsobronchi terminate shortly before the last ramifications of the ventrobronchi. The dorsobronchi therefore do not reach the anterior lateral lung margin (Fig. 23 a–c). They reach the caudal margin of the lung in its lateral part only. The dorsomedial tip of the caudal lung is supplied by the third ventrobronchus. Consequently, the area of lung surface supplied by dorsobronchi is significantly smaller than the area supplied by the ventrobronchi. The dorsobronchi spread only over that part of the lung surface situated cranially in front of the primary bronchus, turning caudally, and dorsal to the posterior primary bronchus. The ventrobronchi on the other hand supply almost the whole ventral lung surface, a variously wide cranial zone of the dorso-lateral surface and their dorsocaudal tip. Corresponding to this arrangement of dorso- and ventrobronchi the lungs of all birds are completely identical, from

headed gull, *Larus ridibundus*, ×1.9. Large saccobronchus into the abdominal air sac (E'), secondary ostia (B''), (C'') lateral to the lung hilus. b) Domestic fowl, *Gallus domesticus*, ×1.4. Secondary ostia (B''), (C'') at the lung margin at the level of the hilus. Ostium into the posterior thoracic air sacs (D') displaced towards caudal. c) Song trush, *Turdus philo-melos*, ×3.2. Ostium of the laterobronchus for the posterior thoracic air sac (D'), completely separated from the saccobronchus (D'') which lies at the lung margin. — *2* primary bronchus, A' ostium for the cervical, B' for the interclavicular, C' for the anterior thoracic, D' for the posterior thoracic, E' for the abdominal air sac penguins to song birds. Only proportional variations exist. In penguins the zone of the dorsolateral lung surface supplied by ventrobronchi is narrow, in loons and grebes very wide.

As in the ventrobronchi, in the dorsobronchi also parabronchi, very close to each other, originate from the dorsobronchial surface directed towards the interior of the lung, passing perpendicularly or obliquely into the lung interior (Figs. 18, 31). In a large number of species, starting from ducks and swans, loons, grebes and auks via fowllike birds and pigeons and plovers, curlews and sandpipers as far as the song birds, parabronchi also originate from the lateral side of the initial portion of the dorsobronchi (Figs. 21a, 22a, 23c, 24c, 25a–c, 26a–c, 30a, b, 32c, 33a–c). They are a part of the parabronchial net between primary bronchus and posterior air sacs, which, if better developed, includes as origin the external side of the initial portion of the dorsobronchi too. Thereby, not only the primary bronchus is shifted into the depth of the lung but also the initial portions of the dorsobronchi. In pigeons, fowllike and song birds the parabronchial net, situated lateral to the primary bronchus extends as far dorsally that it originates from all larger dorsobronchial branches too, and covers their surface (Figs. 25b, c, 26b, c). The dorsobronchi in different avian lungs differ only by the variation of parabronchial origins at their lateral sides. The dorsobronchi are distinguished from the ventrobronchi not only by their very much smaller area of supply but especially by the fact that they do not communicate with an air sac. Neither directly nor indirectly via smaller branches the dorsobronchi open into one of the anterior or posterior air sacs. Thus the dorsobronchi do not only differ from the ventrobronchi but also from the laterobronchi, which will be discussed below. This is true for all birds.

The Laterobronchi

Those secondary bronchi, which originate opposite to the dorsobronchi on the ventral side of the primary bronchus, and pass along the lateral lung side towards ventral, are the laterobronchi. In penguins, cormorants and emus they pass at the lateral lung surface (Figs. 20a, 23a, 24a, 32a). In these species which possess a posterior primary bronchus that is slightly curved towards dorsal, they originate opposite to the anterior and middle dorsobronchi. Their number varies between two, in the emu, and three laterobronchi in penguins and cormorants. In their initial portion the laterobronchi, as the rest of the secondary bronchi, are directed towards cranial to turn towards caudal very soon. An exception is found in penguins in which the initial portions of the laterobronchi take a course directed caudally. The first laterobronchus is the largest, it runs into the posterior thoracic air sac, suddenly dilating after a short, slightly caudally directed course (Figs. 24a, 32a). Only in penguins the first laterobronchus is a small, blindly closed stump (Fig. 32a), the second laterobronchus is responsible for the communication with the posterior thoracic air sac. The one or two remaining laterobronchi branch at the lateral lung surface between primary bronchus and inferior lung margin, thus continuing into the parabronchial net developed in this region, which communicates with the fourth ventrobronchus.

This development of the laterobronchi very clearly characterizes the normal relations of the laterobronchi in all other birds. In these species generally the first, sometimes the second laterobronchus is very well developed. After a short stretch, sharply directed towards cranial, it turns into a caudal direction and with a funnel-shaped dilatation, after a variously long course, it enters the posterior thoracic air sac (Figs. 24 b, c, 26 a–c, 32 b, c, 33 a–c). Only in storks, with their two posterior thoracic air sacs, these are connected to two large laterobronchi, directly following each other (Fig. 32 b). Except in penguins, cormorants and emus, in all other birds the laterobronchi are separated from the lung surface by a parabronchial net (Figs. 23 b, c, 25 a–c). This is also true for that laterobronchus which connects the posterior thoracic air sac, as well as for the remaining one to three laterobronchi. Very shortly after their origin from the primary bronchus they give off parabronchi not only towards the interior of the lung but also towards the lateral lung surface (Figs. 24 b, c, 26 a–c, 32 b, c, 33 a–c).

In the same way, in which a network of parabronchi is interposed between primary bronchus and abdominal air sac, beginning in storks and finding its highest development in fowllike and song birds, an additional connection through a parabronchial net is developed between primary bronchus and posterior thoracic air sac. The parabronchi arise from the lateral side of the initial portion of the posterior primary bronchus and from the large laterobronchus and open into the oblique, laterally dilated opening of the laterobronchus into the air sac. If this additional connection into the posterior thoracic air sac is developed, the parabronchial nets between primary laterobronchus and posterior thoracic air sac and between primary bronchus and abdominal air sac connect to each other, and other parabronchi arising from the rest of the laterobronchi are added (Figs. 23–26, 30 a, b, 32 b, c, 33 a–c, 34 b, c).

The laterobronchus for the posterior thoracic air sac shows a development different from the primary bronchus if the additional parabronchial net between primary and laterobronchus and the thoracic air sacs is well developed. While the primary bronchus becomes increasingly smaller corresponding to the increasing development of arising parabronchi, passing into the abdominal air sac (Fig. 26 b, c), until it cannot be demonstrated as such in song birds, the laterobronchus always remains as a very well developed connection between primary bronchus and posterior thoracic air sac (Figs. 24 a–c, 26 a–c, 32 b, c, 33 a–c). The opening of the parallel parabronchial net into the air sac may become autonomous, this is indicated in loons and fully developed in song birds. Then, the parabronchial ostium into the posterior thoracic air sac lies at the lateral margin of the inferior lung surface, while the ostium of the laterobronchus into this air sac is shifted medially to the middle of the ventral lung surface (Figs. 15, 29 c).

The large laterobronchus that connects to the posterior thoracic air sac and the few other laterobronchi, which give rise to parabronchi into the part of the lung beneath the primary bronchus, lie directly in contact with the lateral lung surface in penguins and cormorants. If they are more and more shifted into the lung interior by the developing parabronchial net which connects the posterior air sacs parallel to the primary and laterobronchus, all other laterobronchi still remain in a plane parallel to the lateral lung surface.

If in large birds the additional parabronchial net for the posterior air sacs is well developed, as in swans, then additional laterobronchi may be found

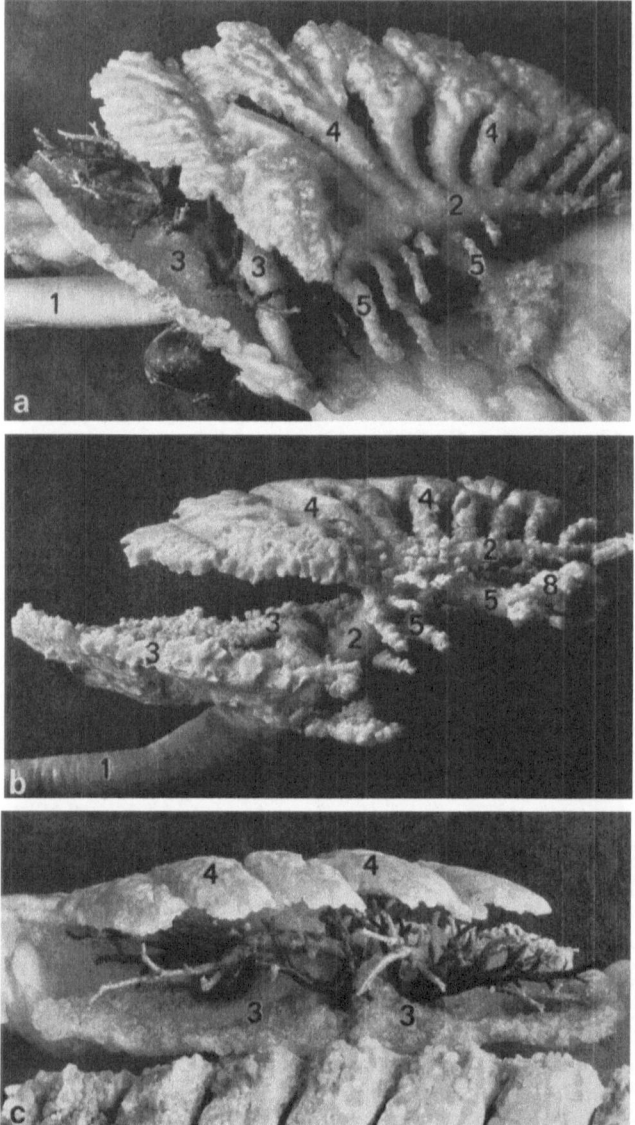

Fig. 30a–c. Mute swan, *Cygnus olor*, injection casts of the left lungs with technovit; primary and secondary bronchi and the vascular tree have been prepared. ×0.5. a) View from lateral on the trachea (*1*) and on the posterior primary bronchus (*2*) with dorsobronchi (*4*) and laterobronchi (*5*). Vessels are visible between dorsobronchi and ventrobronchi (*3*). b) View from lateroventral on the left lung exhibiting the two layers of dorsobronchi (*4*) and ventrobronchi (*3*) which are originating from the primary bronchus (*2*) (sandwich). The parabronchi and the vascular tree between these two layers have been removed. (*8*) saccobronchus into the posterior thoracic air sac. c) View from dorsomedial between the dorsobronchi (*4*) and ventrobronchi (*3*) with the vascular tree. Aa. pulmonales light, Vv. pulmonales dark. Dorsal margin of the right lung with rib incisures at the lower edge of the picture

within the large parabronchial net. They are weaker compared to the original laterobronchi, appear like enlarged parabronchi, differ, however, from these by their larger diameter and in the way they give rise to parabronchi of normal size into all directions. They also do not stand in the plane of the original laterobronchi, but in the middle of the additional parabronchial net (Fig. 30a, b). That is the reason why they do not originate from the ventral side of the primary bronchus but more laterally between the arising parabronchi. They are of variable length, mostly directed towards lateral and caudal. Their number and position may show significant variations among different members of the same species. A variation to such an extent is totally unknown in all other secondary bronchi. The additional laterobronchi are lacking in all smaller birds; in these species only a parabronchial net lateral to the original laterobronchi is developed.

The Saccobronchi

In numerous species, which possess a well developed parabronchial net between primary and laterobronchus and the posterior air sacs, this net does not directly open with its many single parabronchi into the large funnel of the primary and laterobronchus, leading into the air sacs, but the parabronchi accumulate in one, more seldom in a few larger bronchi. These saccobronchi are situated at the inferior lateral lung margin and lateral to the primary and laterobronchus, generally opening into the latter's funnel into the air sac (Figs. 24a–c, 26a–c). The saccobronchi are very differently wide and long, specific for the individual groups of species and related to the size of the lung and the extension of an additional, lateral parabronchial net. Developed best is usually the saccobronchus leading into the abdominal air sac. Often it runs quite a distance at the lateral lung margin, directly beneath the lung surface, collecting the parabronchi, and enters the air sac lateral to the primary bronchus. In this form it is very well developed in auks and plovers, curlews and sandpipers (Figs. 23c, 24c). In auks, this saccobronchus even has a significant number of branches which collect the parabronchi from the dorsal and medial portion of the additional network and enter the saccobronchus in a unipennate manner. In song birds it is equally well developed; because of the reduction of the primary bronchus, however, it opens solely into the abdominal air sac (Figs. 25c, 26c).

The saccobronchus into the posterior thoracic air sac usually is significantly shorter, stump-shaped or developed only as a funnel-shaped orifice, as in cranes, swans, and many other species (Figs. 24b, 26a). In swans the funnel-like orifice may be divided in a few individual, short and wide, cone-shaped saccobronchi (Fig. 30a). These saccobronchi, especially the short ones, are subject to a considerable variation among individuals of one species, as are the additional laterobronchi. The emu possesses a well developed saccobronchus. However, it passes from caudal to cranial, lateral and caudal to the only laterobronchus, the funnel-shaped opening of which, leading into the posterior thoracic air sac, is also the orifice of this saccobronchus. It supplies the inferior portion of the lateral lung that lies beneath the primary bronchus; for this zone further laterobronchi have not been developed.

Branches or parabronchi of the first and second ventrobronchi may accumulate in a funnel-shaped orifice into the additional ostia of the interclavicular and

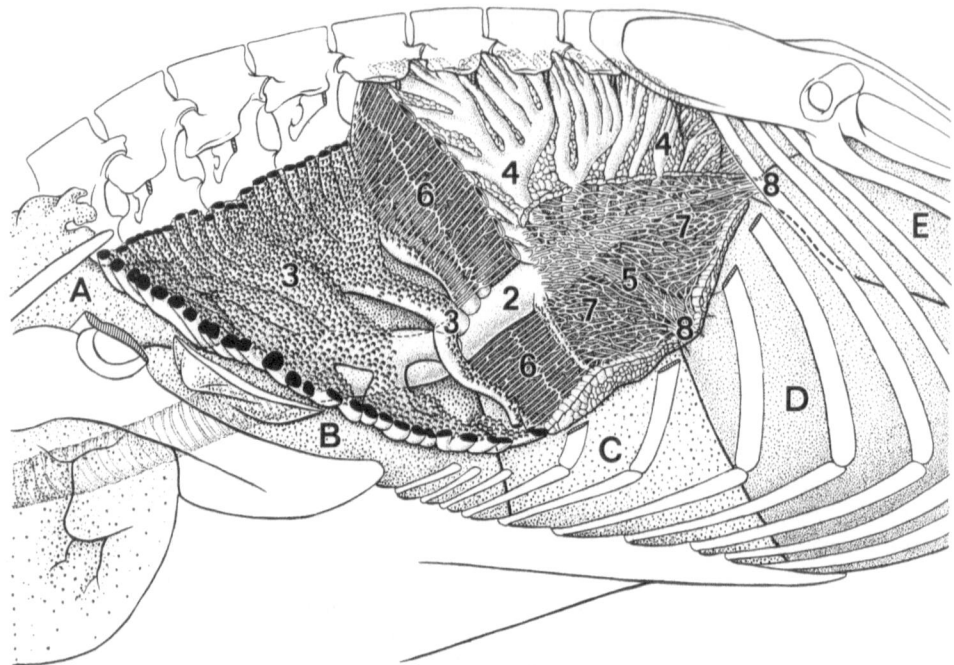

Fig. 31. Semi-schematic drawing of the left lung and its air sac connections of a mute swan, *Cygnus olor*. Anterior portion of the dorsobronchi (*4*) and their parabronchial net (*6*) to the ventrobronchi (*3*) removed; the superficial layer of the thin walled bubbles of the caudo-lateral part of the lung removed, so that the parabronchial net between primary bronchus (*2*) and posterior air sacs and the origins of the dorsobronchi (*4*) and the laterobronchi (*5*) and the openings of the saccobronchi (*8*) into the air sacs are visible. — *A* cervical, *B* interclavicular, *C* anterior, *D* posterior thoracic, *E* abdominal air sac

anterior thoracic air sacs that are situated lateral to the lung hilus in birds. These orifices may be termed as saccobronchi, too. Their extension also markedly varies. Often their orifices are so wide, as in the grey heron (Fig. 21 c), that a bronchial structure cannot be seen. Only seldom are the saccobronchi of the anterior air sacs condensed into short portions which appear as bronchi, as in the chicken (Fig. 29 b).

A denomination as saccobronchus is not correct, if a large branch of the first ventrobronchus, as in the rhea (Fig. 11) or the lateral branch of the second ventrobronchus, as in the stork (Fig. 32 b) opens into the additional ostium of the interclavicular air sac, situated laterally to the lung hilus. These branches of the ventrobronchi then behave similar to the other air sac connecting secondary bronchi. This type of additional air sac connection, in the rhea and stork, is very rare within the class of birds.

A longer saccobronchus, into the abdominal air sac only, is present in auks, plovers, curlews and sandpipers, ducks and song birds (Figs. 23 c, 25 a, c). In auks this saccobronchus even ramifies. Much more often, and typical for the other air sacs, the saccobronchi may be found as short funnel- or cone-shaped

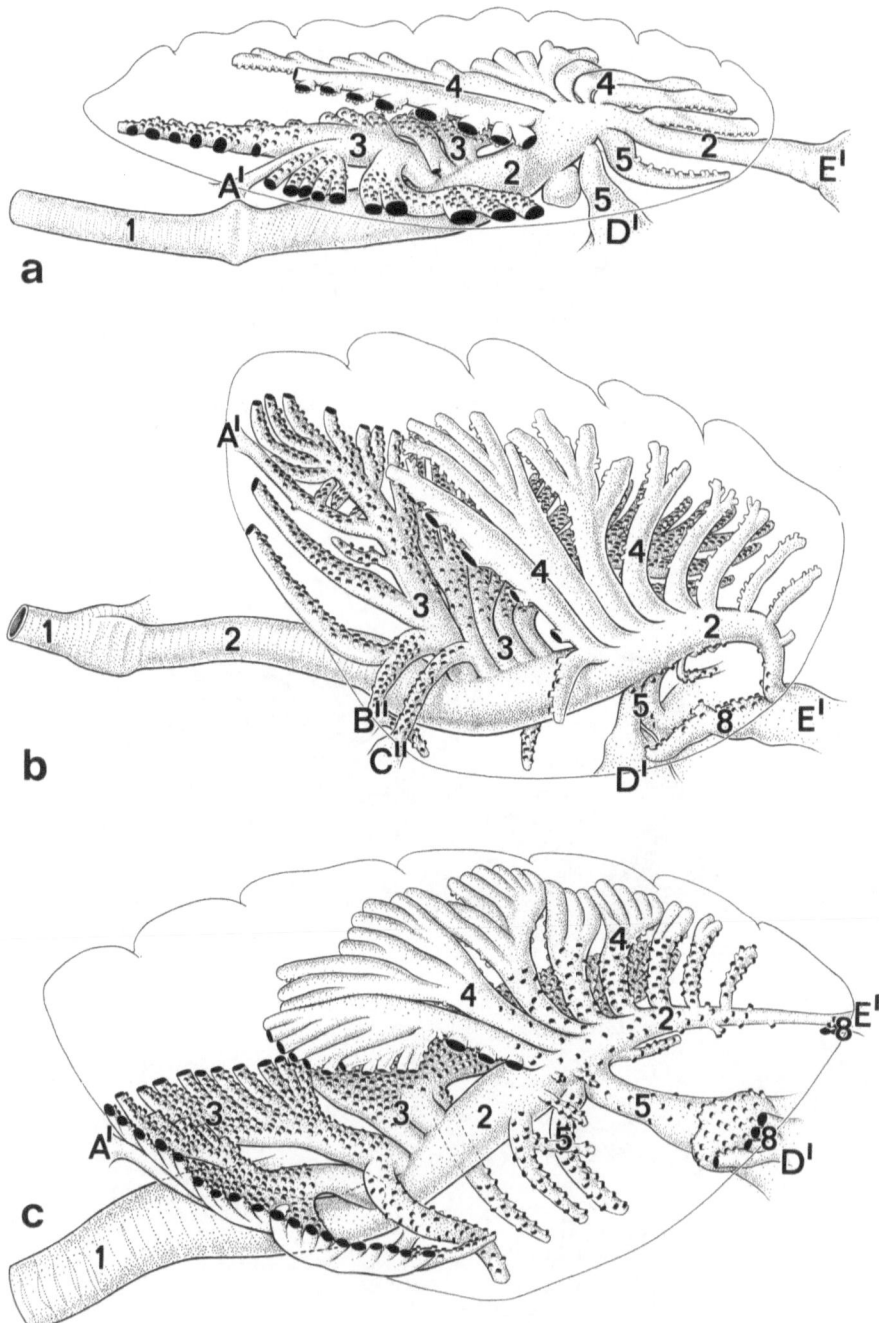

Fig. 32 a–c. Drawings of injection casts of the bronchial system of the left lung seen from lateral. Primary and secondary bronchi have been prepared. a) King penguin, *Aptenodytes patagonica*, ×0.55. b) White stork, *Ciconia ciconia*, ×1.0. c) Mute swan, *Cygnus olor*, ×0.65.— *1* trachea, *2* primary bronchus, *3* ventrobronchi, *4* dorsobronchi, *5* laterobronchi, *8* sacco-bronchi. *A'* ostium into the cervical air sac, *B''* additional ostium into the interclavicular air sac, *C''* additional ostium into the anterior thoracic air sac, *D'* ostium into the posterior thoracic air sac, *E'* ostium into the abdominal air sac

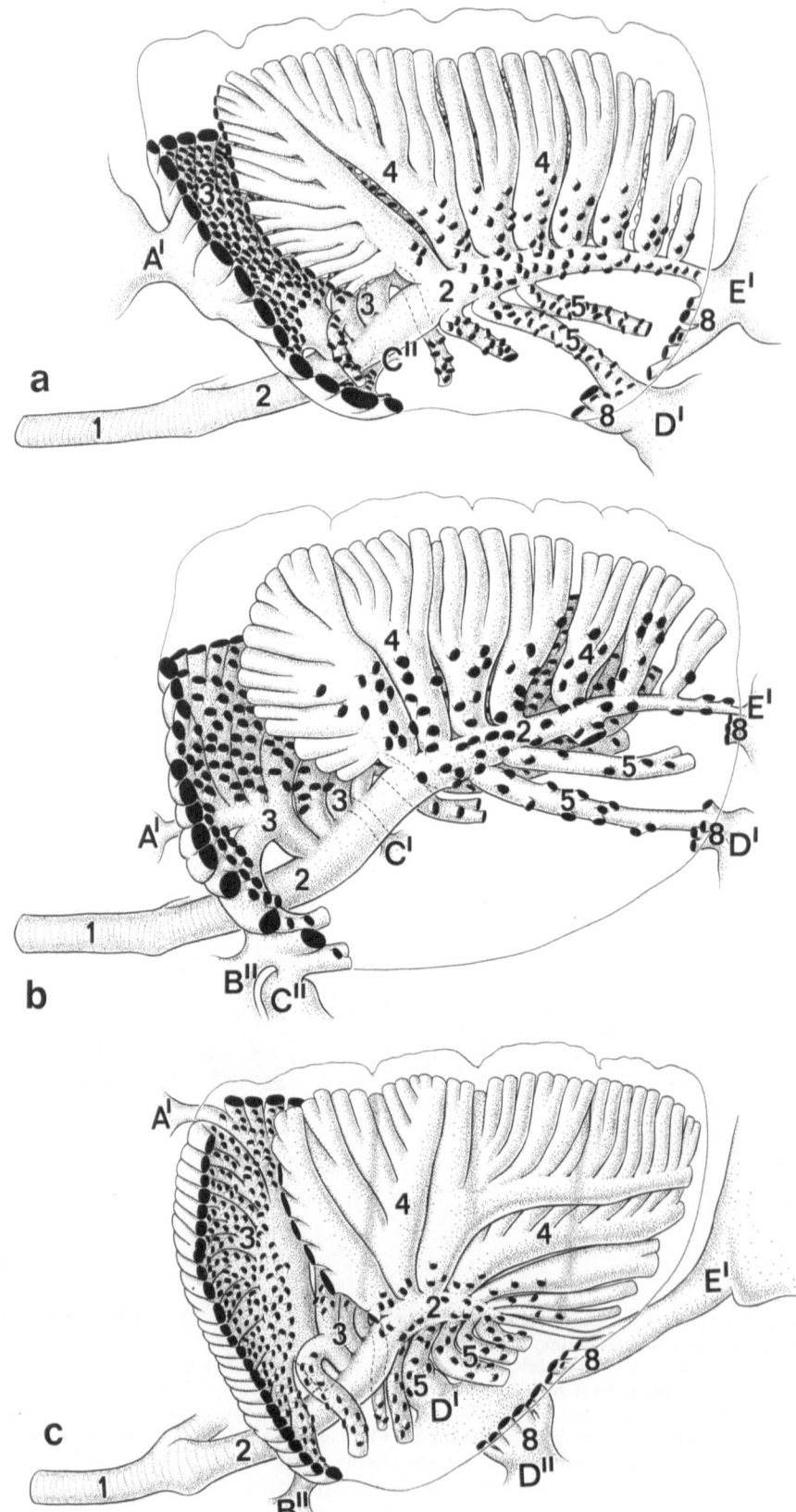

Fig. 33a–c

condensations of the communicating parabronchi. In the additional ostia for the anterior air sacs the saccobronchi are often present as very large orificial zones of numerous parabronchi or small branches of the first ventrobronchi.

III. The Parabronchi

The parabronchi originate, closely beside each other, from the whole surface of the secondary bronchi, directed towards the interior of the lung and their terminal ramifications (Figs. 18, 30a–c, 31). From the sides of the secondary bronchi opposite to each other the parabronchi pass towards each other, to make contact and connect to each other in a medial plane (Figs. 18, 31). They represent the smallest bronchial unit of the avian lung.

The parabronchi are generally characterized in that they have the same size and diameter in all parts of the lung. The diameter is specific to the species but varying to a greater degree from species to species. The smallest observed values, about 0.5 mm, are not underscored even in the smallest birds, like small hummingbirds and goldcrests. The thickest parabronchi with a diameter of about 2.0 mm may be found in birds of very different size, as in the coot, chicken, king penguin and mute swan. Between these values lie the parabronchial diameters in all species investigated. Smaller birds indeed have smaller diameter values and larger birds often greater parabronchi, but the parabronchial width is, beside by body and organ size, determined by the functional capacity of the individual species: good flyers, like common buzzard or old world kestrel have lesser parabronchial diameters than running birds, like chickens and pheasants, always in relation to the same body size.

The parabronchial width, specific to the species, is quite exactly maintained; the variations of diameter make up less than 20% of the corresponding mean value. If variations are present, the thinner parabronchi are found in the lung region around the hilus; they consequently originate from proximal portions of the secondary bronchi, while the wider parabronchi may be found in the peripheral parts of the lung. An exception from the constancy of the parabronchial width specific to the species is found only in penguins. In the king penguin the parabronchi originating from the proximal portions of the secondary bronchi have a diameter of 0.5 to 0.8 mm, while in the periphery of the lung they may reach a diameter of 2.0 mm.

The parabronchi originate from those surfaces of the secondary bronchi, which are directed towards the interior of the lung. The narrow tubes of the parabronchi arise directly from the wide bronchus; the parabronchi retain the same diameter along their whole course (Fig. 35). In part the parabronchi also originate

Fig. 33a–c. Drawings of injection casts of the bronchial system of the left lung seen from lateral. Primary and secondary bronchi have been prepared. a) Common sandpiper, *Tringa hypoleucos*, ×4.5. b) Domestic fowl, *Gallus domesticus*, ×1.7. c) Jackdaw, *Corvus monedula*, ×2.8. — *1* trachea, *2* primary bronchus, *3* ventrobronchi, *4* dorsobronchi, *5* laterobronchi, *8* saccobronchi, *A'* ostium into the cervical air sac, *B''* accessory ostium into the interclavicular air sac, *C'* ostium and *C''* additional ostium into the anterior thoracic air sac, *D'* ostium and *D''* additional ostium of the accessory lateral parabronchial net into the posterior thoracic air sac, *E'* ostium into the abdominal air sac

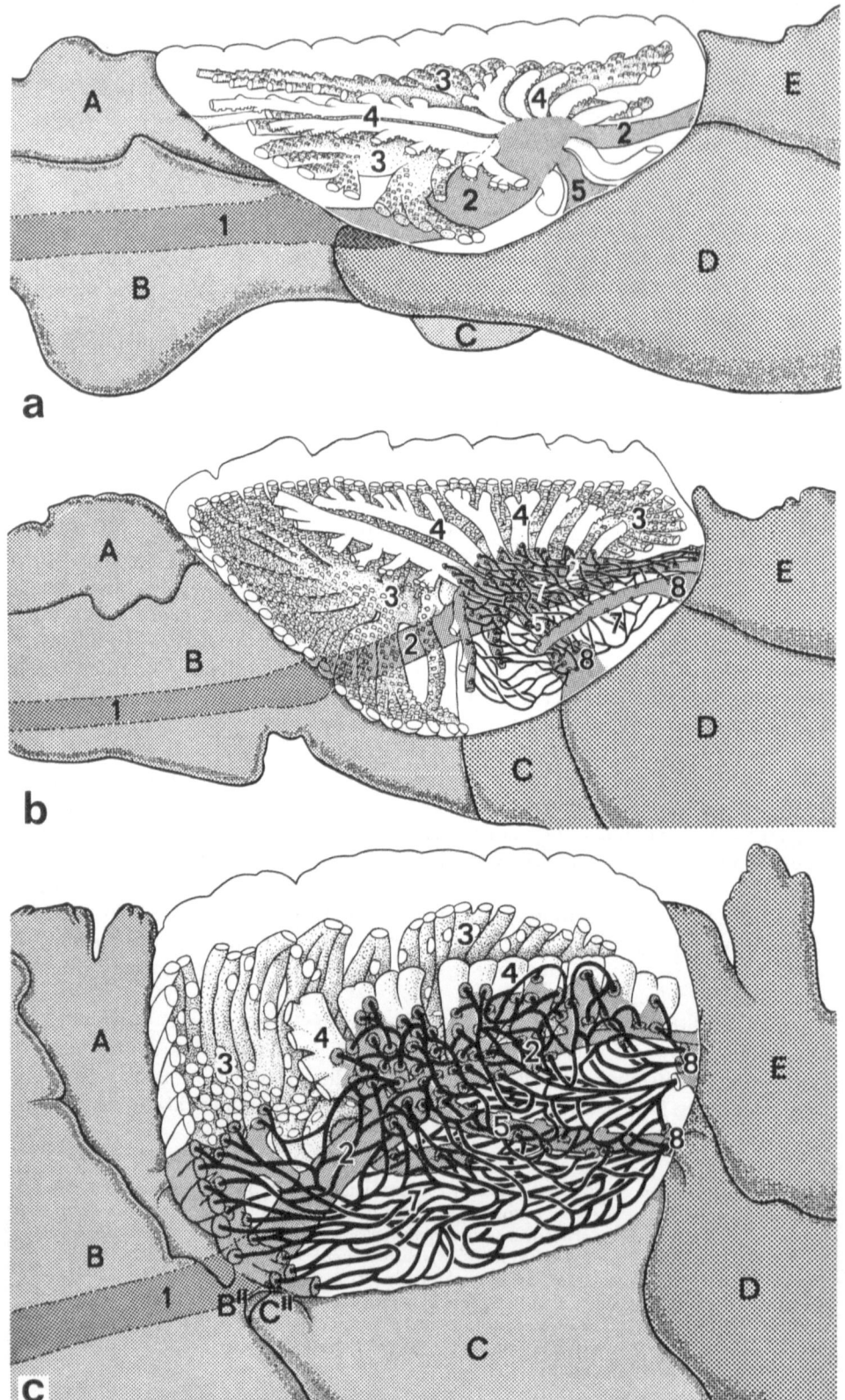

a

b

c

Fig. 34 a–c

from the terminal branchings of the secondary bronchi, which continually taper off into the parabronchi. The parabronchi arising from the ventrobronchi on one side and from the dorsobronchi and laterobronchi on the other side, run towards each other and meet in a medial plane, where they cross link. They form a system of long, parallel tubes which is stretched out between the internal side of the ventrobronchi and the dorsobronchi and laterobronchi, respectively, and which completely fills the space between the two superficial layers of secondary bronchi by its compact accumulation. This huge package of parabronchi, the respiratory tissue of the avian lung, is enclosed like the filling of a sandwich between the two superficial layers of secondary bronchi (Figs. 18, 30b, c, 31).

Within this compact respiratory tissue pass only lung vessels besides parabronchi (Fig. 30a, c). They ramify between the parabronchi, crisscrossing them in right or acute angles, and form a vascular tree, which also lies completely between the two superficial layers of secondary bronchi. Except at the lung hilus, the vessels have no connections at all to the secondary bronchi. They enter and leave at the lung hilus and as larger branches preferentially pass through the parabronchial mass. The vascular tree resembles the mammalian blood vessel distribution in arrangement, ramification and size and thus markedly differs from the highly specialized bronchial system of the avian lung.

A special arrangement of the parabronchial net is found in different parts of the lung for two reasons: 1) The ventrobronchi and the dorsobronchi as well as the laterobronchi are not situated opposite to each other along their whole extension, but the ventrobronchi overlap the dorsobronchi cranially, at the anterior lateral lung margin and dorsocaudally; 2) no ventrobronchi stand opposite to the ventrocaudal portion of laterobronchi. The parabronchi originating from the laterobronchi and dorsobronchi are mainly directed obliquely towards cranial and medial. In the posterior dorsal part of the lung the parabronchi are running directly towards medial or even a little caudal because of the caudal overlapping of the ventrobronchi, while in the inferior ventral part of the lung they are directed sharply towards cranial, in the inferior part towards ventral

Fig. 34a–c. Semi-schematic drawing of the bronchial system and its air sac connections. a) King penguin, *Aptenodytes patagonica*. The posterior air sacs important for the ventilation. are connected only through the primary bronchus (*2*) into the abdominal air sac (*E*) and through the laterobronchus (*5*) into the posterior thoracic air sac (*D*). b) Northern mallard, *Anas platyrhynchos*. The posterior air sacs (*D*) and (*E*) have connections through an accessory lateral parabronchial net (*7*) besides through the primary bronchus (*2*) and the laterobronchus (*5*). The parabronchial net (*7*) originates from the primary bronchus (*2*), the laterobronchi (*5*) and the initial portions of the dorsobronchi (*4*), and leads into the abdominal air sac (*E*) and the posterior thoracic (*D*) air sac, condensed in saccobronchi (*8*). c) Domestic fowl, *Gallus domesticus*. The accessory parabronchial net (*7*) which connects the posterior air sacs (*D*) and (*E*) parallel to the primary bronchus (*2*) and the laterobronchus (*5*), has expanded cranially and occupied the whole lateroinferior portion of the lung. Thereby this accessory parabronchial net communicates with the ventral branch of the first ventrobronchus (*3*) and at the same times relates to the additional ostia (*B''*) into the interclavicular and (*C''*) into the anterior thoracic air sac.—*1* trachea, *2* primary bronchus, *3* ventrobronchi, *4* dorsobronchi, *5* laterobronchi, *7* accessory parabronchial net between primary bronchus, laterobronchi and dorsobronchi and posterior air sacs, *8* its saccobronchi. *A* cervical, *B* interclavicular, *C* anterior thoracic, *D* posterior thoracic, *E* abdominal air sac because of the cranial overlapping of the ventrobronchi. Along this direction of the parabronchial net also it can be shown that the area of parabronchial origin from dorsobronchi and laterobronchi is smaller than that from the ventro-bronchi. The differences in the areas of origin are balanced by branchings or cross linkings of parabronchi. Especially intensive cross linking is found for once directly after their origin from the secondary bronchi and second in the midplane of the sandwich, where the parabronchi, arriving from both sides, do not directly pass into each other but cross link with a few of the opposite side each (Figs. 18, 31).

This compactly arranged network of parabronchi between the ventral and dorsolateral secondary bronchi, therefore has three planes of increased cross linking between each other. Including the special direction of the parabronchial course, the parabronchial system in this form is very constantly found in all birds. Differences besides their width can be found in their total length, which is related to the variable thickness of the lung and in their degree of cross linking. In cranes for instance the parabronchi pass straight and hardly cross linked through the lung, while in swans they are very intensively cross linked along their whole course.

Contrary to the constant extension of this parabronchial net, the network of parabronchi between primary and laterobronchi and the posterior air sacs varies extensively from species to species. In penguins it is totally lacking, in storks, cormorants, cranes and emus (Fig. 23a, b) it is weakly developed, much better already in plovers, ducks and swans (Figs. 23c, 25a), developed to its fullest extent in pigeons, fowllike and song birds (Fig. 25b, c). It originates, if better developed, not only from the primary or laterobronchi but also encroaches on the external side of the initial portions of the dorsobronchi. In pigeons, fowllike and song birds it has incorporated the dorsobronchi to such an extent that even at their peripheral parts they do not reach the lung surface (Fig. 25b, c). This para-bronchial net is always directed towards ventral and caudal, and laterally con-verges into the funnel-shaped orifices of the primary and laterobronchus, or already, shortly before, into the saccobronchi also communicating with the orifice. A very dense cross linking, regularly extended along the whole net, is charac-teristic for this additional network. A striking difference between this and the previously described net between dorsobronchi and ventrobronchi is that the supply vessels pass together with the net, parallel to the direction of the para-bronchi, and do not cross the parabronchi. — In the plane of the original latero-bronchi the two parabronchial nets come into communication with each other. There the parabronchial system between ventrobronchi and dorsobronchi cross links with the parabronchial system between the posterior primary and secondary bronchi and the posterior air sacs. No differences between these two systems can be found in diameter and wall structure of the parabronchi (Fig. 31).

If the dorsobronchi are farther apart, as in storks, the network of the para-bronchi comes to lie directly at the lung surface. This may be observed especially when the additional network is better developed. In pigeons and chickens, the whole laterodorsal lung surface may be occupied by normally developed para-bronchi. In some species a variation of the parabronchial structure may be observed, when they pass directly beneath the lung surface, as in ducks, herons, and flamingos, and markedly in swans (Fig. 8). In these small groups of species all superficial parabronchi dilate into larger, thin walled vesicles, which also may appear like beads on a string. Thus the lung is enclosed into a mantle of thin walled vesicles not only on its laterodorsal but also on its ventromedial surface, which completes the layer of the secondary bronchi. In these species no respiratory tissue at all appears on the surface. Many small air sac diverticula may arise from this system of superficial bubbles and penetrate into the neighbouring bones.

The parabronchi are the smallest units of the bronchial system; they have diameters between 0.5 and 2.0 mm and in their size are specific to the species. Their size shows relations to the body size and functional capacity of the birds. Well flying species have parabronchi narrow compared to running species, large species show wider parabronchi compared to smaller species. The parabronchi are for once stretched out as a parallel system of tubes between the superficial layers of dorsobronchi and ventrobronchi; they arise from the whole inner surface of these secondary bronchi. They cross link, especially at their origin and in the midplane. Another parabronchial network forms an additional connection between primary and laterobronchus, respectively, and the posterior air sacs. This parabronchial system is characterized by its high degree of cross linking, and is not found in all birds. It is lacking in penguins and emus, develops according to the ascending systematic position of the species and is developed to its highest extent in fowllike and song birds.

Wall Structure of the Bronchial System

The trachea is surrounded by skeletal rings on all sides in all birds. These rings are of different configuration in the individual species. Regularly they are broader than the interval between them. They overlap each other like tiles even when the neck is stretched. They are always constructed in the following way: a ring at the right side overlaps the preceding and the following ring, at the left side on the other hand, it lies under the preceding and the following ring. The ring following next behaves just opposite to the preceding. Thus the trachea is completely incompressible even in a stretched state. Narrow parts at the dorsal and ventral sides of the tracheal rings assure the unrestrained tracheal mobility since the rings may slide above each other. These skeletal rings consist of hyaline cartilage, in numerous species, however, they ossify, generally in the region of the syrinx, in many, mostly large species, even along the whole length of the trachea. Often they may be observed as two bony semicircles which are connected to each other by cartilage. In large species, as swans, geese, cranes, and loons, the tracheal rings are completely bony.

The hyaline or bony rings are embedded in a well developed connective tissue, which is differentiated as lamina propria between the tracheal epithelium and the skeletal rings and as tunica adventitia that limits the trachea against the surrounding tissue. The major part of these two connective tissue layers and also of the connective tissue membranes developed between the tracheal rings, consists of collagenous fibers which preferentially pass in the longitudinal direction. Besides, they contain elastic fibers, which are present in the lamina propria to their greatest extent. It is striking that the elastic fibers in the internal elastic marginal layer of the lamina propria are mostly oriented in a longitudinal direction. In the other layers they don't pass in a transverse or longitudinal direction, however, but very regularly in an oblique direction, crossing each other in the form of a right angle and forming a very regular, loose grid that consists of a few fiber layers. This grid very closely spins round the skeletal elements. Smooth muscles are not present in the avian trachea. The striated Mm. sternotracheales and bronchotracheales as well as their differentiations are externally situated on the tunica adventitia.

The inside wall of the trachea is lined by a pseudostratified cylindrical epithelium. In penguins, large round to oval islands of cells which exclusively produce mucus are found in the epithelium. If the intraepithelial glands grow in size, they sink beneath the superficial epithelial layer and form hemispherical to alveolar, partly even tubular, glands which deeply invade the lamina propria but always open towards the epithelial surface. Number and distribution of the glands vary markedly in the different species. The small parakeets have numerous tubular glands, completely under the epithelium, while in song birds the inferior portion of the trachea seems to have a few glands only. Single goblet cells, embedded in the cylindrical epithelium are found in many species, often exclusively, as in some song birds, or together with tubular glands, as in parakeets. However, these relations were not systematically studied in the present work.

In the region of the bifurcation, either a little above, directly in or a little below the bifurcation, the syrinx, the vocal organ of birds, is developed in many avian species. There the development of the tracheal rings has been modified in various manners, specific to the species and family, so that larger membranes or solid cushions of connective tissue, and often muscles are differentiated in this region. Thus the syrinx is a remarkably differentiated, highly diversified organ which possesses a great systematical importance and therefore has often been studied.

I. The Primary Bronchus

After the bifurcation the two primary bronchi are not any more completely surrounded by skeletal elements, but only from the sides with ring parts. These parts have various forms specific to the species, ranging from semicircles to almost complete rings. At the walls opposite to each other, the walls remain membranous. In many ducks (Fig. 19b) the membranous strip is very narrow, in grey herons half the wall is membranous (Fig. 21c). The other species vary between these two extremes. The membranous sheet of the initial portion of the primary bronchus is directed towards medial, at the entrance into the lung hilus it turns more towards ventral. The ring parts of the primary bronchi are usually narrower than the tracheal skeletal rings, and they regularly decrease in width in the interval between the bifurcation and the lung hilus. They continue beyond the lung hilus and extend as very narrow braces as far as to the wall of the vestibulum. In the different species they either completely end already shortly behind the origin of the ventrobronchi, as in song birds and ducks or they lie in the wall of the primary bronchus as far as in the region of the origin of the first dorsobronchi, as for instance in gulls and buzzards.

It is very remarkable that the skeletal ring parts are arranged in the region of the ventrobronchial origin in such a manner that they run through the margin of the thin septum which separates every two ventrobronchial ostia. In the margin of the anterior wall of the first and in the margin of the caudal wall of the fourth ventrobronchus, such braces are also developed. These narrow braces give rise to a perpendicular skeletal spine at the middle of their margin, which, variously far in the different species, ascends into the dividing septa of the ventrobronchi. Not only the anterior margin but also the first portion of the dividing septa is thus supported by a skeletal element. This structure is found very regularly in all species.

On the contrary, the skeletal semirings never show any relation to the ostia of the dorsobronchi and laterobronchi or even to their adjoining walls. While the skeletal rings of trachea and syrinx often ossify completely and always have a well developed medullary cavity, the ring parts of the primary bronchus ossify only incompletely or not at all. They possess either a compact cartilaginous nucleus within a very thin bony lamella or remain totally cartilaginous.

After the bifurcation of the trachea, smooth muscles may be found in the two primary bronchi. They continually cover the membranous wall portion as a thin layer 3 to 8 muscle cells thick. Their fibers run preferentially circular. To a large part they pass in obliquely or longitudinally running bundles, too, which lie on the circular muscle layer on the outside and partly also on the inside. The circularly running fibers pass as bundles between the cartilaginous ring parts, to the perichondrium of which they partly attach. The external, well developed bundles of obliquely and longitudinally running smooth muscles always pass across the outside of the cartilaginous braces. The smooth muscles continue on the primary bronchus, after vanishing of the cartilaginous braces, as a complete, circular muscle layer, from which, both on the inside and the outside, originate oblique and longitudinal muscle bundles. These muscles in the same arrangement around the openings of the secondary bronchi continue on to their initial portions.

The muscles as the skeletal elements lie between lamina propria and tunica adventitia of the primary bronchus. Besides collagenous fibers, elastic fibers also are developed in both layers. However, even in the internal elastic marginal layer of the lamina propria of the primary bronchus they are not arranged in longitudinal fiber bundles, but rather, very regularly, pass obliquely in both directions to the axis of the primary bronchus in all layers. Therefore they cross each other in a right angle and, as a regularly structured grid, surround the primary bronchus, in a more solid lamina propria and a looser tunica adventitia. Both layers closely connect to the skeletal elements, with their fibers passing into the perichondrium. The wall of the primary bronchus is very structured until its abdominal air sac ostium and independent of its diameter. Directly before the funnel-shaped dilatation of the primary bronchus into the ostium of the abdominal air sac, the circular layer of smooth muscles is thickened along a short stretch. In this portion it slowly increases in thickness from cranial, being completely lacking at the initial portion of the dilatation into the ostium. Not only the smooth muscles but also the arrangement and thickness of elastic fibers continue from the primary bronchus on to the initial portions of the secondary bronchi. The parabronchi, on the contrary, originating from the primary bronchus, immediately show their specific wall structure.

The epithelium is a pseudostratified, cylindrical ciliated epithelium along the whole course of the primary bronchus, just as in the trachea. Besides single goblet cells, glands in the form of intraepithelial islands are present. They may be sunk beneath the epithelium as alveolar or tubular glands. The larger glands markedly decrease in number from the syrinx towards the entrance into the lung and further towards the caudal end of the primary bronchus, while the single epithelial goblet cells increase in number. This is for instance true for penguins and ducks, while in parakeets and song birds the total number of glands is small.

This structure of the primary bronchus is principally equal in all species studied. In all species these structure elements are found in the arrangement and distribution discussed above. The largest differences exist in the distribution of epithelial glands. Further variations can be found only in the extent of development of the particular structures. In penguins for instance the wall of the primary bronchus is structured heavy on the whole, especially lamina propria and tunica adventitia are thicker, while ducks have a primary bronchus wall much thinner. In thrushes these structures are so delicate that the epithelium becomes simple cuboideal towards the caudal end of the primary bronchus. These variations of the thickness of the primary bronchus wall do not seem to correlate directly with the body size, for sparrows and budgerigars have a relatively thicker wall with a higher epithelium, compared to thrushes.

II. The Secondary Bronchi

The structure of the primary bronchus wall is continued in the initial portion of the secondary bronchi. Except the openings of the ventrobronchi which are supported by cartilaginous braces directly at their origin (see above), no skeletal elements are existent in their further course. At the marked dilatation, appearing shortly after their origin, the ventrobronchi retain a complete layer of muscles only in a few species, as in penguins and rheas. In these species too, the musculature which is primarily arranged circularly and possesses single oblique or longitudinal fiber bundles, becomes increasingly thinner towards the periphery so that at last it consists of only one layer of muscle fibers. In the secondary bronchial wall directed towards the inside of the lung the layer of muscle fibers diverges around the openings into the parabronchi.

In most of the species in which the ventrobronchial branches lie directly beside each other, the walls of neighbouring branches fuse into a single wall. This is always true for the initial portions of the ventrobronchial branches originating from a ramification and running beside each other. There, the muscle layers ascending or descending from the two external or internal walls of the neighbouring branches mostly fuse into one layer, the external layer of connective tissue disappears completely. In numerous cases even an external layer of muscles, more often the external layer of connective tissue splits off, forming an uninterrupted common membrane across a number of ventrobronchi.

In most other species the smooth muscle layer looses its uninterrupted arrangement shortly behind the origin of the ventrobronchi. Generally, wide, circular bands of muscle fibers remain. These bands are a few, often even only one layer of muscle cells thick. Between the muscle bands, strips devoid of muscles are situated. They are still narrow in the rhea, wider in the swan, and in ducks often wider than the muscle bands. In many species, for instance thrushes, grey herons and gulls (Fig. 21 b, c), rarely narrow, one-layered circular or oblique muscle bands are developed. Whether solid and regular or only as narrow one layered bands, the muscle fibers run crowded between the openings of the parabronchi, partly projecting into the lumen, on that side of the ventrobronchi that is situated towards the lung. Towards distal the development of the muscles always becomes less ordered so that in some species long stretches of the ventrobronchi are devoid of muscles.

The connective tissue of the ventrobronchi is arranged in the same way as in the primary bronchus. Lamina propria and tunica adventitia are thinner, however. Elastic fibers are found beside collagenous fibers mainly arranged in an oblique and right angled pattern, crossing each other and forming a well developed network. The lamina propria always has the better developed network. If muscles are lacking, both networks are united. The epithelium having few glands or none at all, is still prismatic only at the origin of the ventrobronchi. In the further course of the ventrobronchi the epithelium is lower on the bundles of muscle fibers, often only cuboideal, if still ciliated. If the muscles are lacking in the ventrobronchial wall, the epithelium soon becomes flatter and turns into a cuboideal or squamous epithelium.

The wall of the ventrobronchi is constructed in this manner in most species. The ventrobronchi are interrupted on their inside only by the often rather wide openings into the parabronchi (Fig. 35). In individual species the wall structure of the parabronchi with its comparting into atria and the development of respiratory tissue on the inside of the ventrobronchi extends as far as to the lateral ventrobronchial walls, as in some ducks. The comparting into atria is always extended further than the development of respiratory tissue. However, the ventrobronchi are never round about comparted into atria or lined by respiratory tissue.

The ostium of the first ventrobronchus into the cervical air sac is a more or less marked dilatation of a particular branch of this ventrobronchus, which leaves the level of the other ventrobronchial branches towards ventral and penetrates the anterior thin part of the horizontal septum. The wall structure of this branch does not at all differ from the other ventrobronchi; its musculature is at least as far present, as it can be demonstrated as a bronchial branch, slowly and continually tapering off towards distal until it is totally lost. Nowhere along this course a thickening of the mainly circular muscle layers is found. Thus the muscles behave similar to all other ventrobronchial muscles, in most species not forming a closed muscle layer but being divided in individual circular bands. The ostia into the interclavicular and anterior thoracic air sacs, originating from the third ventrobronchus are simple holes in the ventrobronchial wall and the horizontal septum lying underneath. The muscle bundles diverge around them, practically without developing any kind of sphincterial muscles. After penetrating the horizontal septum they immediately dilate to the complete width of the air sacs and then show only the structures of the air sac walls.

7*

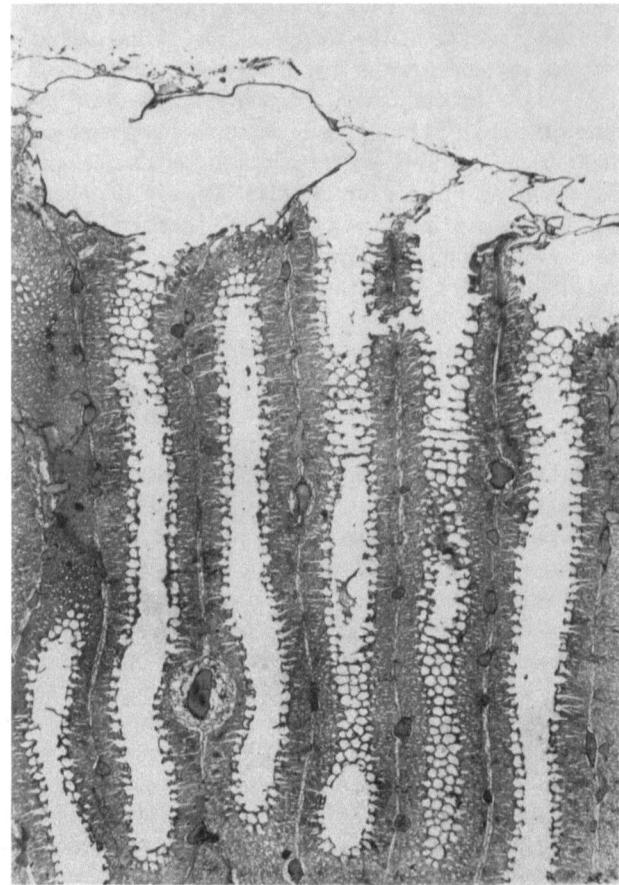

Fig. 35. Lung of a European pochard, *Aythya ferina*, parabronchi in longitudinal section. Bouin, resorcinfuchsin-nuclear fast red, 8 μ, ×20. Thin walled ventrobronchi in cross section. Parabronchi originating from them and separated from each other by septa of connective tissue

The dorsobronchi do not fundamentally differ in their structure from the ventrobronchi. However, they lack supporting skeletal elements even in their initial portions. In the primary bronchus also the skeletal braces at the most reach only as far as to the origin of the first dorsobronchus. The dorsobronchi, contrary to the ventrobronchi, remain independent with their lateral walls, because these don't fuse with each other. The dorsobronchi usually are provided with a better developed muscle layer. The mostly circular musculature, continuing from the primary bronchus on to the wall of the dorsobronchi, reaches as a closed, solid layer far distally. Thus the disintegration of the musculature in individual bands appears further distally as in the ventrobronchi. As in the ventrobronchi and the primary bronchus, marked deviations of the structure, specific to the species, appear in the dorsobronchi, too. If wall and musculature in the primary and ventrobronchi are well developed, as in penguins, they are also well developed in the dorsobronchi. The grey herons on the contrary, and thrushes, having a thin primary bronchus wall and a wide, membranous ventrobronchial wall, containing few muscle cells, have also a weakly developed musculature of the dorsobronchi (Figs. 21a, 22a), which soon separates into muscle bands and larger wall stretches devoid of muscles.

The dorsobronchial lamina propria, with its obliquely running and perpendicularly crossing meshes of elastic fibers, do not substantially differ from the lamina propria of the primary bronchus. The longitudinal fiber bundles are totally lacking in the dorsobronchi. Very similar, only much thinner, is the tunica adventitia. The epithelium in the dorsobronchi is completely identical to the ventrobronchial epithelium. At the initial portions it is still prismatic with numerous goblet cells, at those wall portions devoid of muscles it is only flat and usually not ciliated. Differences, specific to the species, are, of course, found. In some ducks even the flat epithelia are partly ciliated, while in pigeons and thrushes the cuboideal epithelia of the secondary bronchi already are not ciliated. The dorsobronchial walls are structured similar to parabronchi in a larger number of species, the ventrobronchi do not so often show this wall structure.

Then, the musculature is separated into very narrow, circular bundles with large intervals between. Between these bundles the wall is comparted into a number of atria, at the floor of which respiratory tissue may be developed. This transformation of the dorsobronchial wall is not only found in small branches but also in large dorsobronchial stems. In a number of species the development of respiratory tissue is not limited to the inside of the dorsobronchial wall, but lines them round about, equally well developed as in parabronchi. In song birds, pigeons and chickens this is even found as far as to the main stems of the dorsobronchi, partly even very shortly after their origin from the primary bronchus (Figs. 25b, c, 26b, c). Then the dorsobronchi can be distinguished from the parabronchi only by their position, their relation to the primary bronchus and their size, their wall structure is completely identical to the parabronchi's. In the species mentioned above, all branches reaching the dorsolateral lung surface, both parabronchi and dorsobronchi, are on the outside provided with a well developed mantle of respiratory tissue. Such a development is never found in the ventrobronchi, at the most, in the smaller branches at the inside of the lung as far as on to the septa between the individual branches they are supplied with atria; the development of respiratory tissue always has a much lesser extent.

However, in some species, as gulls and buzzards, the dorsobronchi and all parabronchi reaching the surface of the lung are not surrounded by a mantle of respiratory tissue but all secondary and parabronchi reaching the lung surface have only a very thin, membranous wall. This tendency is developed to its fullest extent in swans, in which the whole dorsolateral surface is occupied by thin, vesicular diverticula of the secondary and parabronchi. In this species, the lung is surrounded by a mantle of air vesicles without respiratory tissue on its surface and partly on its ventral side. The membranous vesicles consist of a cuboideal to squamous epithelium and a thin layer of connective tissue with delicate, very thin nets of elastic fibers, corresponding to the air sac walls.

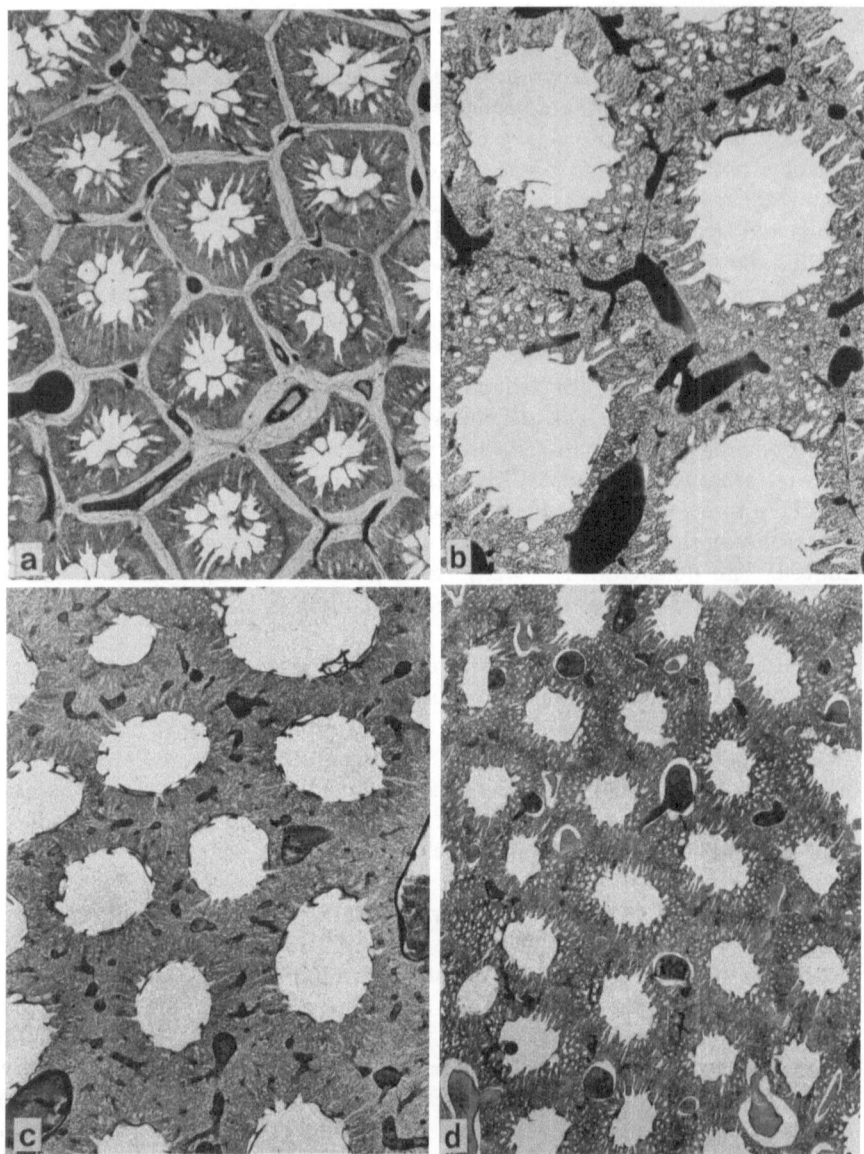

Fig. 36 a–d. Parabronchi of different type and size and with changing proportions of respiratory tissue in cross sections. Bouin, resorcinfuchsin-nuclear fast red, 8 μ, ×23. a) Coot, *Fulica atra*. Basic type of the parabronchi with broad mantle of connective tissue limited by a hexagonal packing. Around the lumen the muscle bands held by the septa which limit the atria. Infundibula issue into the mantle of respiratory tissue. Larger vessels in the mantle of connective tissue. b) Mute swan, *Cygnus olor*. Wide parabronchi with flat atria and septa, very thin mantle of connective tissue around the parabronchi. About 50% of the volume occupied by respiratory tissue. c) Domestic pigeon, *Columba domestica*, narrower parabronchi, low atria and septa and no limiting fibrous septa around the parabronchi. About 65% respiratory tissue of the whole parabronchial volume. d) Budgerigar, *Melopsittacus undulatus*. Highly developed type of the parabronchi. No limiting mantle of connective tissue around the parabronchi and no atria. The respiratory tissue of the parabronchi is continual with the neighbouring, radially penetrated by infundibula. Very narrow parabronchi with about 80% respiratory tissue of the parabronchial volume

The laterobronchi do not differ from the dorsobronchi in their differentiation and in their wall structure. They completely follow the differentiation of the other secondary bronchi specific to the species. In penguins they are provided with a smooth wall having a lot of muscles, in song birds, pigeons and chickens they possess a well developed respiratory tissue which also forms the wall. The accessory laterobronchi, present in particular species, cannot be distinguished from parabronchi by their structure and often by their size. They are marked only by their position and the high degree of ramifying parabronchi.

The first or second large laterobronchus, which connects the posterior thoracic air sac, possesses a closed layer of muscles like the primary bronchus, especially in larger species which do not contain respiratory tissue in the laterobronchus wall. Corresponding to the musculature of the primary bronchus at its transition into the abdominal air sac, the circular musculature also displays an increase in thickness before the funnel-shaped dilatation into the air sac ostium; however, the increase is less than in the primary bronchus. With the penetration of the horizontal septum, often enough already in the funnel, this muscle layer becomes thinner and totally disappears. If numerous parabronchi of the accessory parabronchial net between primary and laterobronchus open into the funnel-shaped dilatation, the decreasing muscle layer diverges around the openings.

The same structure is observed if the parabronchi, collected into saccobronchi, open into this funnel-shaped dilatation of the laterobronchus. Larger saccobronchi, extending for a longer stretch, have a wall structure similar to the corresponding secondary bronchus. Mainly circular muscle layers are found in their walls; this musculature never exceeds the other secondary bronchial musculature in thickness. Sphincterial thickenings of this circular musculature were not found in species with well developed saccobronchi, as northern mallard and lapwing.

The secondary bronchi, consequently, do not fundamentally but only gradually differ from parabronchi in many species. If the wall of the secondary bronchi is provided with atria and respiratory tissue, it is always differentiated in the manner characteristic for the individual species. If the secondary bronchi are provided with respiratory epithelium on all sides, they differ from the parabronchi only by their size, their position and their connections.

III. The Parabronchi

The parabronchi form the stretched net between the insides and the terminal ramifications of the ventrobronchi and the dorsobronchi and laterobronchi, respectively, and also the network between primary and secondary bronchi and posterior air sacs (Figs. 18, 31). The parabronchi are connected to each other by oblique, or transverse, short branches, in a very different manner specific to the species, especially after the origin from the ventrobronchi or dorsobronchi and then again in the midplane, where one parabronchus is always connected to a few opposite parabronchi. The uniformity in size, which can be recognized macroscopically is correspondent to the microscopically uniform structure within the whole lung. They differ from secondary bronchi, in the wall of which exists respiratory tissue only by their size and position. The transition from the secondary bronchi into the parabronchi is fluent in such species, especially at the terminal ramifications of the secondary bronchi which contain respiratory tissue in their walls. Besides, in the majority of species, an abrupt transition from the wide smooth walled secondary bronchi into the parabronchi without a structural transition is observed at the insides of the secondary bronchi (Fig. 35).

Only the penguins make a marked exception from the constancy of para-bronchial width and wall structure. They possess narrower parabronchi in the region around the primary bronchus and wider parabronchi in the periphery of the lung. Even in penguins, though, the structure is uniform within the species. Specificity of structure and size of the parabronchi are so marked that individual species may be identified by these criteria among a larger number of species.

Among these different parabronchi, specific to the species, a basic type may be emphasized. It may be found in penguins, in a few, hardly flying, terrestrial birds, like chickens and pheasants, and in some representatives of water fowl, especially well developed in coots (Figs. 35, 36a, 37). In these species the para-bronchi are separated from each other by very thick bundles of connective tissue. By a regular, hexagonal structure a very dense packing of the parabronchi has been accomplished. In these lamellae of connective tissue pass the blood vessels, the stems of the A. and V. pulmonalis, passing through, and their branches which supply the adjoining parabronchi. In penguins the connective tissue lamel-lae are broadened for the embedding of the significantly increased number of vessels, which is so characteristic for diving vertebrates. On the contrary, in other water birds like ducks and swans, only a very thin lamella of connective tissue is found as the limitation of the parabronchi so that all vessels impress into the mantle of respiratory tissue of the parabronchi (Figs. 35, 36b).

The lumen of the parabronchus is limited by narrow, circular bundles of smooth muscles (Fig. 36a). The bundles are situated in larger, very regular intervals, each bundle being followed by an interval that is four to five times as wide as the muscle bundle (Fig. 35). These rings of smooth muscles continue radially in the form of a thin membrane, in a plane perpendicular to the para-bronchial axis (Fig. 35). The muscle rings and the horizontal septa are connected to each other by numerous, longitudinally oriented and radial, narrow, and thin septa, more seldom the muscle rings split and run towards the neighbouring bundles (Fig. 37). Thus, a zone made up of relatively large and deep spaces, which communicate with the lumen through a rectangular opening, originates around the central, free lumen of the parabronchus. Henceforth, these spaces will be called "atria" referring to Makowski (1938a) (Fig. 37). The parabronchial atria are separated from each other by thin septa on all sides and at the superior and inferior margin of their openings into the lumen they possess a torus of circular muscle bundles. In this basic type of parabronchi the free lumen is enclosed by a very wide space comparted into atria. Such a parabronchial struc-ture resembles very much a ductus alveolaris of mammalian lungs (Fig. 37).

From the outside of each atrium a number of canals originate regularly; they ramify and give rise to further branches and, decreasing in size, penetrate the dense tissue that surrounds the lumen of the parabronchus. The canals begin with a funnel-shaped invagination of the atrial floor, and decrease from a 50–100 μ diameter to air capillary size (Figs. 36a, 37). The canals are termed "infundibula" referring to King, Ellis, and Watts (1967) in the following discussion. Their initial portions together with the flat atria of the pigeon, have been named "vestibulum" by Krause (1922). The air capillaries, which interlace in all directions with each other, forming a dense network, originate at all levels from the infundibula (Fig. 37). The net of air capillaries is so densely interlaced with the similarly structured net of the blood capillaries that the one net system just fills the interstices of the other net. This interlaced air-blood-capillary net, in which only infundibula are found besides the capillaries, represents the actual respiratory tissue, which forms the mantle of the parabronchi and in which the gas exchange takes place (Figs. 36a, 37). The air capillary net has an unambiguous alignment with the infundibula feeding it and passing radially from the atria into the periphery, from the parabronchial lumen to the periphery of the parabronchus. The blood capillary net is oppositely directed, arising directly at the periphery from the smaller arterioles which are lying in the connective tissue lamellae. The blood capillary net which is, just as the air capillary net, structured in three dimensions, is directed strictly radially from its origin to the center of the parabronchus. At the parabronchial lumen the capillaries then continue into venules which are situated in the wall of the respiratory tissue, directly beneath the roots of the transverse septa dividing the atria. Single branches of these collecting venules penetrate the mantle of respiratory tissue, without collecting further capillaries, and open into veins that lie between the parabronchi (Fig. 37).

The bundles of circular muscles, which limit the free parabronchial lumen together with the anterior margins of the longitudinally oriented septa like a meshy network, are covered by a cuboideal to flat epithelium which is not ciliated. The septa are on both sides covered by a flat epithelium, which has only a little connective tissue between, so that the mesothelium-like epithelium is the substantial part of the septa. This flat epithelium extends as far as into the infundibula, where it ceases to be demonstrable light microscopically. Only rarely small vessels or capillaries are found in the septa, which probably regularly pass to the circular muscle bundles.

Around the muscle bundles, beneath the cuboideal epithelium, a loose but well developed net of elastic fibers is found which spins the muscle bundles in a criss-cross manner and continues as a delicate elastic fiber net into the septa. In the septa too, obliquely crossing fibers dominate. These fine elastic nets end in a network which directly adjoins the mantle of respiratory tissue at the basis of the atria. From this basal network, as well as from the nets of the septa, delicate elastic fibers pass directly underneath the thin epithelium into the initial portions of the infundibula. In the respiratory tissue itself, elastic fibers are never found. Not until the border between respiratory tissue and surrounding connective tissue lamella separating the parabronchus a thin layer of obliquely passing and crossing elastic fibers are observed, while the lamella of connective tissue itself contains very little elastic elements. Each parabronchus is therefore surrounded by a very delicate, adventitial stocking of elastic fibers.

The basic type of parabronchi is only found in birds flying poorly or not at all. Most species flying better and longer do not any more possess a fibrous limitation of their parabronchi against each other, so that the air capillary nets of neighbouring parabronchi change into each other (Figs. 36d, 38). Then, only the

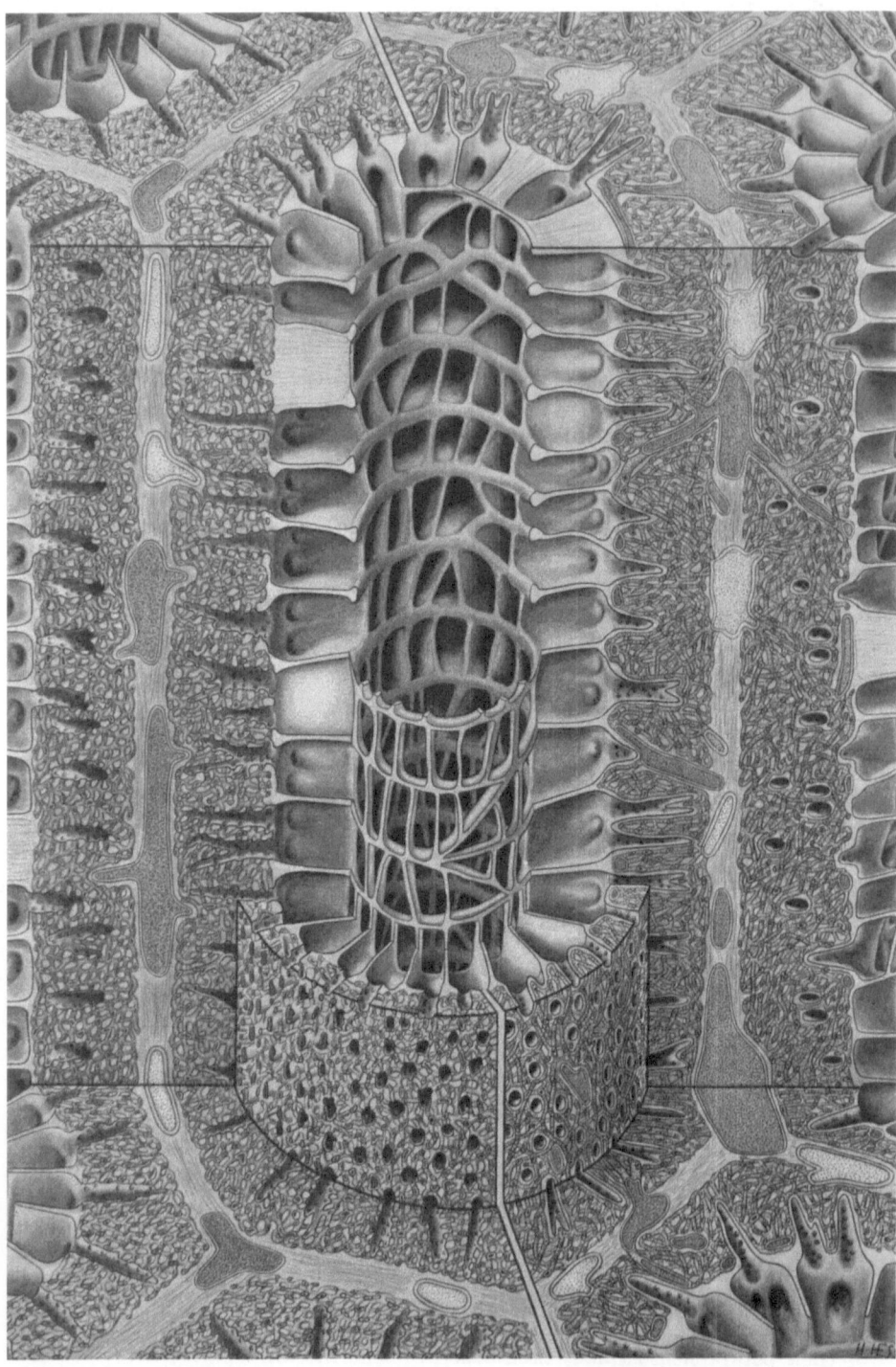

Fig. 37

position of the larger vessels identifies the border between the individual para-bronchial units. Thereby a communication between neighbouring parabronchial lumina exists via the air capillary nets. This continual communication of the parabronchi exists in most birds, from the procellariids and cormorants up to the song birds.

The total diameter of the parabronchi and the thickness of the respiratory tissue mantle deviates significantly from species to species. Accordingly, the volume share of the respiratory tissue in relation to the total lung volume is strikingly changed. The mute swan, king penguin and the chicken possess very large parabronchi—the maximal diameter found in all species studied was 2 mm—and a thin mantle of respiratory tissue with a large free lumen and well developed atria (Fig. 36b). In these species the respiratory tissue occupies only about 50% of the parabronchial and thus of the lung volume. More often narrower para-bronchi with a thicker respiratory tissue mantle are found, making up about 65% of the lung volume. These relations are found in ducks, pigeons, gulls and buzzards which therefore take a middle position in this series (Fig. 36c). At the top of this series of development of respiratory tissue stand the small song birds and parakeets with a very small parabronchial lumen and a very large tissue mantle, which occupies about 80% of the lung volume (Fig. 36d). Not only the share of respiratory tissue in relation to the total lung volume is subject to changes, specific to the species, but also the width of the air capillaries. The air capillaries are very wide in penguins, swans and coots where they have a diameter of about 10 μ, while the smallest air capillaries with a diameter of about 3 μ are found in song birds.

In the deviation of the parabronchial structure, not only the total diameter decreases and the mantle of the respiratory tissue increases in such a manner that its total share of the lung volume rises, but also the atria become increasingly flatter, their septa continually lower, in this sequence of increasing respiratory tissue. Therefore the system of circular bundles of smooth muscles finally lays itself more or less directly on the mantle of respiratory tissue. Consequently, the atria are almost completely abolished, the muscle bundles have usually become thinner (Figs. 36d, 38). Besides the reduction of the atria nothing is changed in the parabronchial structure, even the loose nets of elastic fibers are present in correspondent manner. They spin around the muscle bundles, lie close to the mantle of respiratory tissue and run into the initial portions of the infundibula, where they terminate. Such a maximal development of the re-

Fig. 37. Semi-schematic drawing of the basic type of parabronchi as it can be found in the penguin or in the coot. The free lumen is limited by mostly circular bundles of smooth muscle cells. The zone of the atria follows. Generally a few infundibula pass from the atria into the mantle of respiratory tissue. As is demonstrated on the left side of the scheme, they give rise to air capillaries at all levels which then cross link and interlace. In the interstices of this net lies the blood capillary net which is demonstrated on the right side of the drawing, and which is intensively meshed with the air capillary net. The blood capillary net is supplied by the (light) arteries which lie in the connective tissue lamella that separates the individual parabronchi from each other. Mainly it flows out of the (dark) veins which collect the capillaries directly at the parabronchial lumen

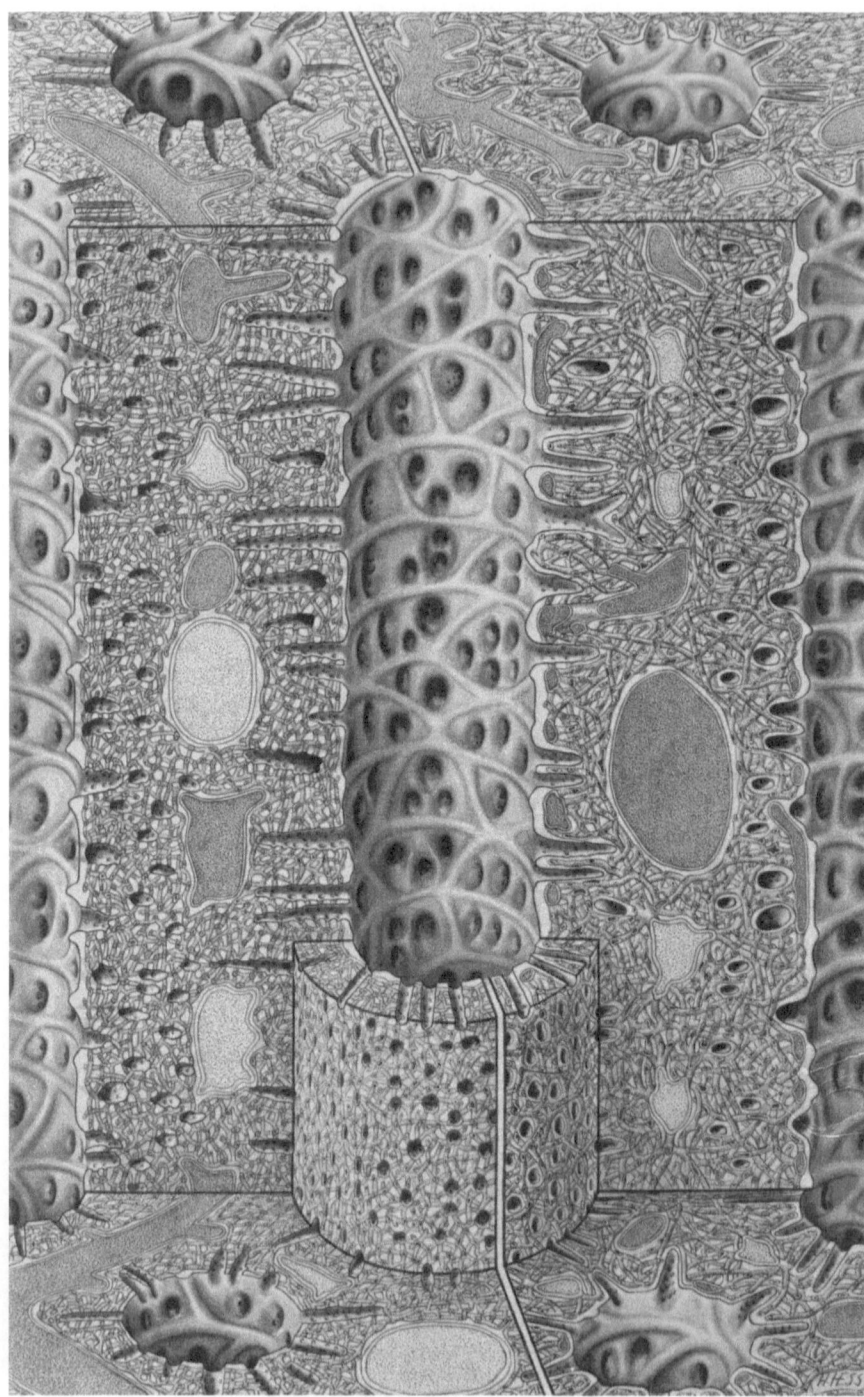

Fig. 38

spiratory tissue and the parabronchi, is already shown in pigeons and then especially small song birds and small parakeets. All other types studied arrange themselves into a series of sliding deviation between the basic type of the parabronchial construction found in penguins and coots and the highly developed type in pigeons and small parakeets and song birds.

Wall Structure of the Air Sacs

The walls of the air sacs in their structure completely correspond to those very thin parts or sections of the secondary bronchi free of muscles. The air sacs are lined by a flat epithelium. It is still relatively high in penguins, almost cuboideal; in the other species it is lower, yet mostly not as flat as an endothelium. This epithelium, if it is not pathologically changed, is always smooth as a mirror. Underneath the epithelium a very thin lamella of connective tissue is situated, which contains a regular, loose net of elastic fibers besides loose collagenous fibers. Usually this elastic net is formed by fibers out of three directions which intersect at an angle of about 60°. The network is of a striking uniformity in the different air sacs and at different points of them. However, this structure is not specific to the air sac walls, for it can be shown that the thin lamella of connective tissue under the peritoneal epithelium on the mesentery or on the septa between liver and intestinal tract has the same structured, loose network of elastic fibers.

The structure of the air sac epithelium with its connective tissue is not influenced by the structures on which it is situated. Usually the air sac walls are grown together with other structures, for instance with the horizontal and the oblique septa, with the body wall and the pericardium, with trachea, esophagus, vessels and nerves. Special relations are found only, when two air sacs enclose very little connective tissue and form a thin membrane, separating the two air sacs, as between anterior and posterior thoracic air sac and between abdominal air sac and wall of the peritoneal cavity. Air sac and peritoneal epithelia, touching each other, form a membrane which has a certain thickness and solidity because of incorporated connective tissue in penguins, rheas and loons. In these and in all other species muscle cells are completely lacking. In higher species this wall is usually so thin that it cannot be demonstrated without injuries when it is prepared from their loose attachments on and between the intestinal convolutions.

Fig. 38. Semi-schematic drawing of the highly developed type of parabronchi which is characteristic for song birds. The atria have been almost completely reduced, the free lumen borders directly on the respiratory tissue on which thin, generally circular bundles of smooth muscles are situated. Infundibula originate between them which give rise to air capillaries at all levels as is shown on the left side. The air capillaries cross link and interlace, and also the air capillaries of neighbouring parabronchi do so, only the vessels mark the former separating border. The blood capillaries, shown on the right side of the drawing, show a behaviour similar to that of the basic type, they originate from the (light) arteries at the border between different parabronchial units and flow out through the (dark) veins, which lie directly at the parabronchial lumen

The extremely thin connective tissue has between both epithelial layers a very loose net of randomly oriented collagenous fibers and a regular net of crossing elastic fibers. It is developed rather regularly in all species and independent of the total thickness of the connective tissue with its share of collagenous fibers. The elastic net of the relatively solid wall of the abdominal air sac in penguins and rheas does not differ from the elastic net of the thinner air sac wall of the other birds or of the delicate membranes of the abdominal air sacs in song birds. This finding indicates that the walls of the air sacs are not subject to an elastic tension, as for instance the avian skin (Petry, 1951). If the membranes are a little thicker because of their increased content of collagenous fibers, they are erected more or less rigid, even in the living condition, while the thin membranes without suspension connect adhesively to each other, or to other structures.

Besides collagenous and elastic fibers the thin connective tissue of the air sac walls contains single vessels originating in the corresponding region. They are well demarcated in those spots where the air sac walls lie on structures with very few vessels, like the horizontal and oblique septa, or where the walls touch each other and form the membranes described above. These very long vessels split into a few capillaries passing very far from each other. Thus, larger regions devoid of any vessels are constructed, especially in the abdominal air sac wall. A general increase of the vessels is only observed when the air sac walls are infected. At particular points, small very flat and mostly oval isles of adipose cells may be found accompanying the blood vessels in some species as for instance in the northern mallard. These islands are distinct already by their rich supply with blood vessels. More often variously large islands of very densely packed nuclei, which probably are flat lymph follicles, are situated along the vessels. They were often found in the mute swan, northern mallard and coot. In some specimens of these species one may find cells filled with anthracotic pigment situated in the periphery of these lymph follicles: macrophages. This pigmentation is striking only in the walls of the posterior air sacs.

Structure of the Horizontal and the Oblique Septum

These septa are very similar to the pericardium in their structure and their nature. In spite of their insignificant thickness they are very coarse and most of all resistant to tension. The bundles of collagenous fibers are oriented according to this characteristic. In the horizontal septum they pass mainly in a transverse direction, from the body wall to the attachment at the vertebral bodies. The fiber course splits around the air sac ostia, completed by fiber bundles running oblique and transverse to the transverse axis. The Mm. costopulmonales are interposed into the course of the transversely oriented fiber bundles at the body wall (Figs. 7a, b, 11, 13, 15, 16a–h, 17a–h), also splitting around the particular ostia and forming one side around the cranial and the other side around the caudal margin of the ostium. The bulk of the collagenous fibers, passing through the oblique septa, runs fan-like from the M. tensor septi obliqui towards the sternal margin and the ventral abdominal wall and issues cranially into the pericardium (Fig. 11). Additionally, collagenous fibers originate from the dorsal attachment at the vertebral bodies in front of the M. tensor septi obliqui. They run towards ventral, also fanning out towards cranial and caudal. In the caudal part of the oblique septum also fiber tracts of different directions superpose on the main bundle which originates from the M. tensor septi obliqui. They arise dorsal to the abdominal wall and run obliquely or perpendicularly towards ventral again entering the abdominal wall. Additionally, fibers of the septum separating the liver from the abdominal cavity, issue into the oblique septum.

In almost all birds muscle fibers besides the well defined M. tensor septi obliqui are not existent in the oblique septum. Contrary to the striated Mm. costopulmonales, the M. tensor septi obliqui consists of smooth muscles. The muscle bundles dispersed in the oblique septa of penguins and rheas, occasionally also in chickens and swans, also are consistent of smooth muscles. In these species the muscle fiber bundles which can be found ventral to this muscle in the oblique septum, are arranged in random directions. Additionally, muscle fibers also appear in the septum between mesentery and left oblique septum which adjoins the gizzard, and issue into the oblique septum. Origin and insertion of all fibers and the muscles of the trunk wall is the fascia thoracica interna or its caudal continuation, respectively, the fascia transversalis. Additionally, in the thoracic region the two septa, especially the horizontal with its Mm. costopulmonales, attach to the ribs. In the caudal region of the oblique septum, a portion of the abdominal musculature may be split and incorporated into the septum in large birds, for instance in swans.

The two septa contain almost no elastic fibers. Smaller bundles of elastic fibers appear only between the muscle fibers of the Mm. costopulmonales and tensor septi obliqui. Otherwise only the delicate elastic nets which belong to the connective tissue of the air sac and peritoneal epithelia are found on these septa. They are immediately attached to the septa, unless the septa are grown together with other organs, as the horizontal septum on its dorsal side with the lung, or the oblique septum on the right side with the vena cava caudalis and a part of the liver. At those points, where the oblique septum attaches to the sternum via more or less numerous tissue bridges, and where oblique or horizontal septum attach to the trunk wall via slight folds or small septa, or where such small folds are constructed between the two septa or between these and the membranes separating the air sacs, the connective tissue of the superposed air sac wall is altered. At these points, the fine elastic network is not anymore developed in the regularity usually found, but there the elastic fibers are straightened and concentrated along the direction of the tissue bridges or folds. Thus the elastic fiberwork of the air sac wall behaves in a manner similar to the lamina propria of the secondary bronchi around the bronchial invaginations of their wall and mostly around the muscle fiber bundles which are variously wide and project from the wall in the formation of atria.—Vessels are also rare in the horizontal and oblique septa, they often pass in interstices between the larger collagenous fiber bundles.

Discussion

The Avian Lung as a System of Mostly Rigid Tubes

The development of joints between bodies and transverse processes of the thoracic vertebrae and the two widely separated capitula of the ribs, fixes the

axis for the rib motions. The axis stands perpendicular to the vertebral column
for the first ribs and is shifted towards caudal for the caudally following ribs
so that the first ribs make a pure forward motion about their axis, while the
caudal ribs add a caudally increasing component of an outward motion to the
forward movements (Zimmer, 1935). This outward motion increases for the
individual rib from its portion near the vertebral joint, where it is practically
equal to zero, continually towards the intercostal joint. This mechanism of the
thorax is substantially identical for all types of the avian body, differences are
only found in the proportions and thus in the extent of the individual components of the motion.

The space in which the lungs are enclosed is closed ventrally by the horizontal septum. It is developed as a solid aponeurosis and always stretched tightly
without any folds so that its designation as pulmonary aponeurosis by Huxley
(1882) is easily understandable. It originates medial to the membranous septum
which is often supported by hypapophyses and which forms the medial limit
of the lung cavity together with the narrow high vertebral bodies. This median,
perpendicular septum is tightly stretched by the hypapophyses or only by the
horizontal septa originating from its inferior margin which pass slightly towards
ventrolateral. The lateral attachment of the horizontal septum is characterized
by the fact that it follows the first or the first two free vertebral ribs, to attach
to the first and second or the first to third true thoracic ribs, a little above their
intercostal joints. Here, the horizontal septum has reached its deepest ventral
point, in that part of the thorax in which the ribs make a true forward motion.
The attachment to the following ribs always takes place a little further dorsally
so that the horizontal septum withdraws from that region in which the ribs have
an increasing component of motion towards forward and outward. Caudally, the
horizontal septum terminates with its lamella running towards dorsal variously
far in front of or beneath the ilium.

In this manner, a space is limited by the vertebral column and the perpendicular septum, the dorsal part of the thoracic wall and the horizontal septum
which is subject to only minimal changes in volume during motions of the thorax.
Its special configuration with the lateral deepest point above the first intercostal
joint follows from the principle of maximal utilization of the immobil space;
another fact can be explained by this principle: the shift of the axis for the rib
motions far into this space, unknown in all other vertebrates. Consequently,
the ribs cut deeply into this space and subdivide its dorsal portion in individual
compartments lying between the ribs. Thus, it is accomplished that only the
inferior limitation — the horizontal septum — in its lateral portion experiences a
certain displacement towards cranial during the thorax motions. However, for
this purpose, too, the horizontal septum is attached in a line of optimal conditions,
since the forward component of the rib movement increases also from cranial
towards caudal and since the caudal ribs have an increasing additional outward
component in their motion. The septum with its attachment is shifted more and
more towards dorsal, thus avoiding the region of increasing rib mobility.

It follows that the lung which totally occupies the dorsal thoracic cavity
and has grown together with it at all sides, owes its special configuration to
the principle of minimal change in volume. When it was concluded from the

placement of the lung between the dorsal portions of the ribs that a great change in volume was thus effected (Soum, 1896; Scharnke, 1938), then the mechanism of avian thorax motions had been completely misunderstood, for just the opposite is true. — The horizontal septum has the Mm. costopulmonales in its marginal zone, often enough also a M. sternopulmonalis from the processus anterior of the sternum. These muscles, varying considerably in their width and solidity, are constantly existent and have the effect of stretching the horizontal septum. Of very special importance is the observation of Soum (1896) which was confirmed by electromyographical studies by Fedde, Burger, and Kitchell (1964c), De Wet, Fedde, and Kitchell (1967) that these muscles contract during expiration. Thereby they compensate for the small changes in volume still present, for with their relaxation during inspiration the horizontal septum may remain a little behind during the insignificant downward motion of its lateral attachment, and during expiration it is maintained in its former position by the contraction of the Mm. costopulmonales.

The lung is therefore built into the thorax and limited by the surrounding wall regions in such a manner that it experiences only minimal changes in volume during motions of the thorax. Thus its configuration is determined: Additionally, the Mm. costopulmonales with their contraction during expiration (Soum, 1896; Fedde, Burger, and Kitchell, 1964c; De Wet, Fedde, and Kitchell, 1967) take care of at least partly compensating the changes in volume still existent. Under these mechanical and physiological conditions the lung experiences only in its ventrolateral part a slight shift forward during inspiration.

The cavum pulmonale is maintained practically constant in volume during these respiratory motions. The type of construction of the avian thorax proves to be very resistant to passive deformations, too. The reasons for this resistance are the development of the ribs and the sternum together with the vertebral column which is hardly mobil or partially grown together. The ribs possess fixed axes of motion with their articulations at the vertebral bodies and transverse processes, and with an axis of articulation fixed at the sternal margin by broad joints in the same direction. Arc-like strutting the dorsal thoracic cavity and having a solid articulation at the intercostal joints, they provide for a transverse incompressibility of the thorax. The strutting of the ribs through the dorsal thorax is best developed in well flying species, the arc-like ribs of which originate very deep from the vertebral bodies and cut very far towards ventral into the lungs. This type of construction of the avian thorax is markedly contrasting to that of the thorax of reptiles and mammals in which the ribs are cartilaginously articulated with the sternum so that the thorax is very elastically compressible in all directions.

The constancy in volume of the cavum pulmonale and therefore of the lung grown together with it at all sides has numerous consequences for its internal structure. The lung with all its parts is stretched out in this cavity in such a manner that the strongly changed structure of the secondary bronchi follows immediately. It is striking that the dorsobronchi and especially the ventrobronchi are so thin walled in most species that they contain no muscles at all throughout more or less large stretches. Skeletal elements are never found in their wall, they always terminate at the vestibulum of the primary bronchus. Therefore the dorsobronchi and ventrobronchi are so thin walled that they would collapse at once without the stretching that is caused by the fusion of the lung at all sides. The individual branches of the ventrobronchi usually even do not possess a separating septum of their own but a common septum. Their very thin wall, adjoined to the horizontal septum, covers many ventrobronchi lying beside each other as an uninterrupted membrane which is grown together with the stiff septum so closely that a separation by preparatory means becomes extremely difficult.

Because of the tight attachment and the thin walls of the ventrobronchi which usually have substantially reduced the musculature, variations in their diameter must be excluded. Variations in diameter at constant lung volume could only be effected by a dilatation of neighbouring structures. But since the ventrobronchi are tightly grown together with the horizontal septum at their ventral walls, the possibility of their contraction does not exist. The dorsobronchi are similarly structured and the same is true for their distal, thin walled portions lying directly at the lung surface.

The primary bronchus on the other hand possesses muscles and in its initial portion skeletal elements, too, which allow its comparison with a mammalian bronchus. It may be concluded from its position and its wall structure that the primary bronchus may very well show variations in its diameter even if to a limited extent only. This is especially true for the last portion of the primary bronchus as well as for the great laterobronchus which both display an increase of their circular muscles before their entrance into the posterior air sacs. Since the initial portions of the dorsobronchi are provided with muscles in the same way as the primary bronchus, they also have the ability for a certain variation in diameter, especially in their initial, thin portion of origin. Contrary to these are the initial portions of the ventrobronchi. They always originate from that portion of the primary bronchus that is provided with cartilage and possess hardly any muscles beside the cartilaginous elements in the very thin lips at their origin and the laterally adjoining wall portions. These openings are invariably stretched by their construction.

The cross linked, mainly parallelly oriented tube system of parabronch extends between the two series of ventrobronchi and dorsobronchi lying at the lung surface. Connected to the mainly rigid tubes of the dorsobronchi and ventro-bronchi, the parabronchi as a system of tubes in a lung of constant volume are also invariable in their volume. This is exclusively true only for the mantle of respiratory tissue of each parabronchus of an intimate network of air and blood capillaries.

The air capillaries possess an osmiophilic film on their very thin epithelium, as do the alveoles of the mammalian lung (De Groodt, Sebruyns, and Lagasse 1960; Bargmann and Knoop 1961; Policard, Collet, and Martin 1962; Tyler and Pangborn, 1964; Petrik, 1967; Petrik and Riedel, 1968a, b; Lambson and Cohn, 1968; Akester, 1970; Clements, Nellenbogen, and Trahan, 1970; Macdonald, 1970) which consists of phospholipids (Fujiwara, Adams, Nozaki, and Detmer, 1970). These phospholipids do not differ from those found in the mammalian lung (Pattle, 1958, 1963, 1965; Schoedel and Rüfer, 1968; Scarpelli, 1968). The phospholipids in the alveoles of the mammalian lung decrease the surface tension of water at the constantly moist limiting surface tissue—air to such an extent that an unfolding is possible by muscular forces of the organism, as at birth. If this surfactant is lacking, an unfolding of the alveoles becomes impossible and the new born infant cannot breathe, if the surface film is destroyed later on, the alveoles collapse and the lung becomes atelectatic (Schoedel and Rüfer, 1968; Scarpelli, 1968). These relations are probably the same for all mammals. The smallest alveolar diameters, measured in mammals, have values of 35–40 μ (Tenney and Remmers, 1963; Spells, 1968); thereby the surface tensions must be sufficiently reduced by their surfactant.

The air capillaries of birds have a diameter of only 3–10 μ (Oppel, 1905; Stanislaus, 1937) which is never exceeded according to the author's observations. Pattle and Hopkinson (1963) suggest: "In the bird, collapse of the lung may in part be prevented by its more rigid structure; to prevent transudation, however, a surface film is even more necessary than in the mammal, because the curvature of the walls of the air capillaries of the bird is even sharper than that of the walls of the mammalian alveoli". A rough estimation shows that the surface tension in the air capillaries because of their small diameter is so great, resulting from the sharp curvature, that even a well developed surface film would never suffice to lower the tension to such a degree that an unfolding by muscular forces would become possible (Schoedel and Rüfer, personal communication). It follows that air capillaries are only able to exist as rigid and stiffly stretched structures. The lung volume, constant during all phases of respiration because of the construction of the cavum pulmonale, is therefore a necessary requirement for the development of air capillaries. If the lung volume varied they would collapse and could not be unfolded again. The film of phospholipids, present in the air capillaries has to reduce the surface tension to such an extent that a transudation out of the blood capillaries cannot take place and the air capillaries remain filled with air and do not close by swelling.

The parabronchial mantle of air and blood capillaries is rigid, but the circular muscles which generally are connected with the parabronchial mantle by the thin septa containing elastic fibers, have the ability to dilate and contract without influencing the rigid mantle. Muscles and elastic fibers in the circular bundles and the elastic nets in the septa are the means which are responsible for a continual tension of all elements which is existent in all states of contraction. Characteristically, the rigid mantle of respiratory tissue does not contain elastic fibers (Duncker, 1969), as also King, Ellis, and Watts (1967) proved for the chicken. A contraction of the circular muscles was demonstrated for individual cases by Zeuthen (1942) and for the chicken by King and Cowie (1968, 1969) and Cowie and King (1969). Thereby a good possibility of varying the diameter of the free lumen is given and thus of regulating the perfusion with respiratory air. The complete occlusion of the parabronchi by contraction of the circular muscles, as King and Cowie (1969) observed in vitro, should only be possible for the completely extirpated lung with unlimited mobility. The complete occlusion of the atria, observed in vivo by King and Cowie (1969) also, is probably not possible in the unviolated lung but was made possible by the greater mobility occurring with the opening of the lung which was necessary for the observation.

8*

In the unviolated lung the construction of the circular muscles with the surrounding elastic fibers and the elastic septa between the atria may effect a greater variation of the diameter of the parabronchial lumen and at the same time a change in the width of the atria arising from the parabronchial lumen. An occlusion of the lumen and the atria is not possible in an intact, stretched lung. The relations are different in those parabronchi in which the circular muscles lie directly on the mantle of the respiratory tissue because of the reduction of atria and septa, as in song birds and small parakeets. Here the possibility of contraction and variation of diameter is probably very limited.

Elastic fibers are therefore present in the wall of the primary and secondary bronchi, in the delicate network of elastic fibers around the muscle bundles of the parabronchi, in their septa and directly on the inside of the mantle of respiratory tissue. Besides, those parabronchi which possess a fibrous limitation, have a net of elastic fibers in this separating lamella. Together with the existent smooth muscles these elastic systems serve to keep the whole lung stretched to a certain extent so that all bronchi may be maximally unfolded and that the air capillaries cannot collapse. This may well be observed during the preparation of a living lung, which contracts to about 80–90% of its former volume, after it has been detached from its fusions at all sides; the form of the lung, however, is exactly maintained, not considering the collapse of the thin walled secondary bronchi. The avian lung never collapses to the extent known from mammalian lungs.

If the structure of the bronchi and their arrangement within the volume constant lung is summarized, if follows that the secondary bronchi are rigid tubes, as the parabronchi when viewed as a whole. Additionally, the parabronchi have efficient regulators of their lumen in their circular muscles which are carried by thin elastic septa. Their mantle with the air capillaries always remains rigid. The secondary bronchi do not have any possibility of varying their diameter because of their arrangement within the lung. Contrary to the secondary bronchi, the primary bronchus is probably capable of varying its diameter to a limited extent which, however, is important for the regulation of the air flow. The capability of such variations are surely also existent in the initial portions of the dorsobronchi. The thin muscle bundles, randomly oriented in the other portions of the secondary bronchi, and the nets consisting of characteristically oblique and rectangular, crossing elastic fibers, probably are responsible for the stretching of the thin bronchial walls and thus of the whole lung. In the rigid tube system of the bronchi in the lung constant volume, the primary bronchus and the parabronchi, because of their anatomical structure, are capable of varying their diameters. Thereby the principle of the rigid tube construction is not at all influenced, however, an efficient possibility of influencing the air flow exists.

In the lungs of penguins and rheas the secondary bronchi are provided with a thicker mantle of muscles, the construction principle of rigid tubes is not influenced, however. The ventrobronchi, because of their rigid arrangement in the ventral lung surface and their fusion with the horizontal septum, are not capable of varying their diameter, even in penguins and rheas. In these species, perhaps explicable by their systematic position, the adaptation of the structure of the secondary bronchi to their functional capabilities has probably not been completed totally. In the other species of birds the structure of the thin walled secondary bronchi shows a complete adaptation to a lung of constant volume as a mainly rigid tube system.

The differently well developed saccobronchi are structured identical to the other secondary bronchi. If at all present and not only representing an invagination of terminating parabronchi, they are developed with very thin walls containing elastic nets and sparse muscles, corresponding to the secondary bronchi of their species. The presence of circular muscles was repeatedly postulated at their points of penetration through the horizontal septum and at the openings of primary and secondary bronchi into the air sacs (Eberth, 1863; Fischer, 1905; Schulze, 1910). In exact investigations of this matter, it was found that the Mm. costopulmonales border both the cranial and caudal margin of the ostia lying at the lung margin, best developed at the ostium of the laterobronchus and saccobronchus into the posterior thoracic air sac. The same may be found to a varying extent at the secondary ostia into the interclavicular and the anterior thoracic air sac. The ostium into the abdominal air sac is lined in its cranial margin by muscle bundles from the thoracic wall. All kinds of muscle fiber thickenings are lacking in the ostia into the cervical, interclavicular and anterior thoracic air sacs which are situated in the horizontal septum, in song birds also in the medial ostium into the posterior thoracic air sac.

Arrangement and function of the fibers of the Mm. costopulmonales around the air sac ostia and their contraction during expiration (Soum, 1896; Fedde, Burger, and Kitchell, 1964c; De Wet, Fedde, and Kitchell, 1967) show very clearly that they pull the ostia apart and keep them extended during expiration by stretching the horizontal septum. They can never close the ostia. In the lung of constant volume the bronchi are not only stretched out as rigid tubes but the openings of the bronchi into the air sacs are kept open during all phases of respiration.

Only the wall muscles of the primary bronchus opening into the abdominal sac, partly also the muscles of the large laterobronchus opening into the posterior thoracic air sac show a swelling in the last stretch before the funnel-shaped dilatation. Thus a marked possibility of regulation of the bronchial diameter before its air sac entrance is given. In the variously present saccobronchi a swelling of the thin muscle layer has never been found as yet.

The Posterior Air Sacs as Ventilators of the Tube System

The air sacs must be divided in two groups both according to their position and especially evident according to their connections to the bronchial system. The anterior group, which includes the cervical, the impar interclavicular and the anterior thoracic air sacs, is connected to the ventrobronchi. The cervical sac originates, more or less far cranially, from the first, and the other two from the third ventrobronchus near its origin from the primary bronchus. Besides, the interclavicular and anterior thoracic air sacs possess additional ostia at the lateral inferior surface of the lung (Figs. 28a, b, 29a–c) which have a variable extension, though (Juillet, 1912a). These ostia usually lead directly into the parabronchial net which is developed in the region of the first and second ventrobronchus. Only in a few species, in storks and rheas, a larger branch of the second ventrobronchus opens into the interclavicular air sac, lateral to the lung hilus.

The morphological homogeneousness of this group of air sacs is underscored by the fact that in song birds the anterior thoracic air sacs which are markedly reduced in size, form wide communications with the interclavicular air sac thus uniting. A communication between anterior and posterior thoracic air sac cannot be demonstrated in any species, their separation is absolute. The position of the separating membrane between these two air sacs, may strikingly vary; the anterior thoracic air sac may be very large and extended far toward caudal, as in storks or swans, or reduced to extremely small size, as in song birds.

The posterior group is formed by the posterior thoracic and the abdominal air sacs. The posterior thoracic air sac is connected to a generally large laterobronchus, the abdominal air sac to the primary bronchus, both communicating with the posterior portion of the bronchial system. In the majority of avian species, additional openings into the accessory parabronchial net lateral to the primary bronchus which often are united to a saccobronchus, are added lateral in the wide, funnel-shaped ostia. In song birds the saccobronchus is completely separated from the laterobronchus lying further towards the middle of the inferior lung surface (Figs. 15, 29c). These posterior air sacs are the largest of the avian body. Their connection to the bronchial system is uniform even if the posterior thoracic sac is divided in two sacs, each receiving a laterobronchus. Posterior thoracic and abdominal air sacs markedly differ in their position, especially in relation to the oblique septum, however.

The posterior thoracic air sac, as all air sacs of the anterior group, is situated in front of and dorsal to the oblique septum in the cavum subpulmonale (Huxley, 1882). The abdominal air sac, however, lies behind the oblique septum in the abdominal cavity, in its caudal portion, above or even between the intestinal convolutions. Only the heart and the liver by the post-hepatic septum (Poole, 1909) are separated from this abdominal cavity. Presence and distribution of an abdominal air sac in *Apteryx* are not clear according to the description of Huxley (1882). In all species studied by the author the abdominal air sac behind the oblique septum is well developed, primary and saccobronchus entering it, passing through the dorsal lamella of the caudal horizontal septum into the abdominal cavity, the cavum cardio-abdominale. It is a remarkable phenomenon that, in reference to Huxley (1882), the difference in position and extension of the abdominal compared to the other air sacs is not emphasized in the literature. In penguins and rheas the abdominal air sacs are of limited size and have a coarse wall, in the other species studied, however, they have a thin wall and always such a size that one of them alone is capable of filling the whole abdominal cavity (Figs. 11–17).

The physiological changes in volume of the air sacs, are generated by the respiratory motions, as Zimmer (1935) has exactly analysed basing on the anatomical structure and on the registration of the body movements. Electromyographical investigations of the individual respiratory muscles (Fedde, Burger, and Kitchell, 1964a, c; De Wet, Fedde, and Kitchell, 1967) very exactly confirm the actions of the muscles which had earlier been deducted from the mechanism of the thorax. During the respiratory excursions the ventral thoracic and abdominal wall with the sternum moves against the vertebral column in such a manner that they depart from and approach the vertebral column around a center of motion in the region of the shoulder joint. These movements are rendered possible by the joints of the ribs and the action of their musculature. The sternum with its cranial end does not experience a lowering against the vertebral column, but only a slight forward shift while the caudal end of the sternum is markedly lowered. In the anterior region of the thorax the ribs perform a pure forward motion, while towards caudal they have an increasing component of an outward motion; this outwardly directed movement is greatest in the plane of the inter-costal joints. During inspiration the thoracoabdominal cavity increases both in its dorsoventral and transverse diameter. In the region of the cranial sternal margin this increase is still zero, at the caudal end of the sternum it is maximal. For the transverse diameter the region of maximal dilatation is situated even further towards the caudal end, where the ribs reach far towards caudal.

These motions are fundamentally the same in the terrestrial and swimming forms of the avian body which show only proportional differences. The skeletal elements reaching further caudally in the trunk wall of the swimming type give the abdomen the capability to increase its active motions; this possibility of an increased dilatational movement is compensated by the gravity on the freely mobil viscera in terrestrial birds. Thus differences are found in the major support of the skeletal system during the inspirational motions; in the swimming type vertebral column and pelvis must be lifted against the ventral thoracic and abdominal wall lying on them, in the terrestrial type sternum and abdominal wall must be lowered and lifted against the pelvis resting on the legs together with the vertebral column. In the swimming type the inspiratory part of the respiratory movements must be carried out against gravity, in the terrestrial type the expiratory part (Zimmer, 1935; Stolpe and Zimmer, 1959). It is charac-teristic that the mainly flying species, like gulls, terns and procellariids represent an intermediary type in the construction of the trunk wall. During flight, as during swimming, the body rests on the sternum, consequently, the dorsum must be lifted against gravity during inspiration.

The inspirational motions of the rib cage with vertebral column and sternum are performed by the Mm. intercostales externi with the aid of the Mm. levatores costarum, interappendiculares, costocoracoideus and costosternalis, scalenus and teres. Very characteristic developments of the avian thorax are the processus uncinati of the vertebral ribs, which are otherwise only found in sphenodon and crocodiles. As Zimmer conclusively demonstrated (1935), they are special points of origin for those parts of the Mm. intercostales externi which are mostly termed as Mm. appendicocostales. The processus uncinati are the expression of a highly differentiated and efficient musculature for the inspiration. Developed to their fullest extent are the uncinate processes in diving birds in which they usually reach up as far as the second consecutive rib. This underlines their func-tion in a striking manner, for the animals diving in the expirational position must inspire especially deep and against gravity when they surface.

The motions of expiration are initiated by the Mm. intercostales interni. They are aided and almost completely carried out by all the abdominal muscles. This was found by Zimmer (1935) and electromyographically confirmed by

De Wet, Fedde, and Kitchell (1967). The expiration musculature is of a far greater importance in birds than in mammals, since in a rigidly extended lung and in inelastic air sac walls the expiration, too, must be carried out completely active. The active expiration has been demonstrated by Burkart and Bucher (1961), Wick and Bucher (1963). They were able to show that the first phase is performed by the intercostal muscles, the following strong second phase by the abdominal muscles.

The excursions of the trunk during inspiration and expiration, increasing from cranial towards caudal, involve very different changes in volume for the individual air sacs. The interclavicular sac and the cervical air sacs which may be neglected in this discussion, experience only a very slight dilatation during inspiration. A more distinct dilatation is already found in the anterior thoracic air sac, especially when the latter is large as in storks and swans. The following posterior thoracic air sac has the greatest change in volume of the air sacs lying in the cavum subpulmonale.

For the estimation of the variation of volume of the thoracic air sacs not only the motion of the trunk wall but also that of the oblique septum must be considered. At maximal inspiration the oblique septum will be straightly extended between its dorsal origin and its ventral attachment to the body wall. Since the oblique septum is rigid and inelastic because of its structure and since the small muscle in its dorsal portion has only a limited action, the septum will press into the cavum subpulmonale during maximal expiration and thus aid the diminution of the posterior thoracic air sac. In its posterior part, caudal to the lung margin, the oblique septum may lay itself largely on the trunk wall. In the anterior portions of the cavum subpulmonale a considerable residual volume remains for the posterior thoracic air sac under these conditions. The abdominal sac is the only air sac to lie behind and ventromedial to the septum obliquum. This is of great functional importance. The abdominal air sac, unlike the anterior air sacs, is not always unfolded but is suspended from its dorsal field of fusion as extremely thin sac into the abdominal cavity, above and lateral to the intestinal convolutions, partly between them (Figs. 9–17). Functionally the abdominal air sac is characterized by the fact that in many birds, especially in small species, it may be immensely dilated, but also completely compressed and empty (Stanislaus, 1937). It is the only air sac that has no dead space in small birds.

The air sacs lying in the cavum subpulmonale are not impaired in their unfolding and function by a supine positioning of the bird, since the tightly stretched oblique septum separates them from the mobil viscera. On the contrary, the abdominal air sacs are compressed by the viscera sinking dorsally or at least strangulated at their initial portions. Thereby it becomes intelligible that a bird does not take the supine position physiologically, contrary to a mammal. Quite a few physiological studies have been performed on birds in the supine position, however, often it was not even directly stated. In these experiments true physiological respiration cannot be described, as King and Payne (1964) have shown.

The following may summarize the previous discussion. The dead space of the cervical and interclavicular air sac is large and they are capable of only a very small ventilation; anterior and posterior thoracic air sac display a more significant ventilation, also having a dead space, while the abdominal air sac, at least in smaller species, does not have a dead space, thus being capable of full ventilation. Consequently the importance of the posterior air sacs for the lung ventilation follows. Considering the connection of the posterior thoracic and the abdominal air sacs to the large bronchi of the posterior lung and their large extension found in all birds, the posterior air sacs constitute the bellows which effect the air exchange through the lung.

The lesser participation of the anterior air sacs in this function, especially of the interclavicular sac, also follows from their structure. They differ from the posterior bellows in that a large number of structures, esophagus and trachea, vessels and nerves, additionally numerous thin membranes which compart the lumen, pass through their lumen making impossible large variations in volume. If the interclavicular air sac expands on the sternum towards caudal, ventral to heart and liver, as in large birds like swans and storks, or in song birds, this diverticulum is invaded by numerous coarse tissue bridges which effect the attachment of pericard and oblique septum to the sternum, at the same time rendering impossible variations in volume. These structures are always lacking in the posterior air sacs.

Not considering this functional differentiation which corresponds to the extent of the ventilation of the individual sac, they behave fundamentally identical in inspiration and expiration. This has been proved by numerous pressure measurements within the individual air sacs which have been performed during the individual phases of respiration (Baer, 1896; Soum, 1896; Francois-Franck, 1906; Victorow, 1909). During inspiration the same negative values against the surrounding air pressure appear in all air sacs, and during expiration the same positive values. This is well understandable because of the communication of all air sacs via wide bronchi with the primary bronchus. The whole thoraco-abdominal cavity acts as pressure chamber for the ventilation of the respiratory apparatus, the trunk wall generating the motion. Since the oblique septum with its small amount of muscles is not capable of performing greater actions, not only a homologue of the diaphragm but also an analogue to it is lacking in birds. Their trunk cavity is not, as in mammals, separated in a thoracic and an abdominal cavity by a diaphragm.

It follows from the differences of the position and extension of the anterior and the abdominal air sacs that Perrault (1676), Sappey (1847) and many others were able to observe an antagonistic function of the air sacs when the abdomen was opened. They did not know the functional uniformity of the avian body cavity. A true antagonistic filling may be observed only in air sac parts lying outside the thoracoabdominal cavity, as in a large interclavicular air sac which far overlaps the clavicles (Stanislaus and Böhme, 1938). For the latter's configuration a number of other factors are of great importance: filling of the crop, tension of the M. constrictor colli, extension or bending of the neck etc. Considering the size of the air sac system such factors could probably impair the normal physiological sequence of respiration, but still be neglected. The capacity of the avian respiratory apparatus is so great that it may compensate enormous increases of the dead space of the trachea, which may appear in the large intra- or substernal and subpectoral tracheal loops of some swans, cranes and birds of paradise (Gadow, 1891; Berndt and Meise, 1959) seemingly without any recognizable changes.

The avian lung is a rigidly extended tube system of constant volume which has no elastic distensibility. The walls of the abdominal air sacs contain so little elastic fibers that they, too, cannot generate elastic tension. All other air sac walls are grown together with the wall of the cavum subpulmonale, thus becoming completely passive structures. Only the trunk wall is actively mobil and has an elastic distensibility. This is clearly shown in the first study of the total compliance of the respiratory tract (Scheid and Piiper, 1969). It is still unknown as yet, how the elastic resting position of the thoracoabdominal wall, the respiratory resting position and the normal tonus of the trunk wall musculature are related to each other.

The relations between position, connection and ventilation of the air sacs are the same in all birds. Only in relation to the abdominal air sac most of the large differ from the small birds. While the small species may completely empty their abdominal air sac by compression (Stanislaus, 1937) most of the large birds lack this characteristic. In these species the viscera occupy only a small space of the cavum cardioabdominale so that they do not completely fill this space even at maximal expiration (Fig. 16a–h). Therefore their abdominal sac also has a large dead space. In these large species the other air sacs are also enlarged so that their residual volume has risen, for instance the diverticula between heart and liver and the sternum. This enlargement of the air sac spaces has only a small functional importance for the respiratory apparatus. Because of the enlargement, however, the bird may increase its locomotor system to a greater extent than necessary for its total body weight. In the mammal the weight increases with the third power of length when the organism grows. The same would be true for birds, however, the surface of the wings necessary for flight and the physiological cross section of the flight muscles can only be increased with the second power. The capability of developing large air sacs allows a greater increase of the locomotor system and therefore an extension of the upper size limit for species capable of flying. The increase of the posterior air sacs, especially the abdominal, in large birds thus represents a special type of pneumatisation for the enlargement of the locomotor system and thereby for the maintenance of the capability of flying. In the course of this development the dead space volume of the abdominal air sac very soon exceeds the ventilation volume of this sac.

Zimmer (1935), in his analysis of the avian locomotor system, has proved that the portion for the respiratory movements functions completely independent of the wing muscles. This is confirmed and emphasized for the musculature of the legs also, in the present study. The regular development of the processus uncinati of the vertebral ribs is of important evidence in this connection, too. Since the wing musculature with its functional limitation to wing motions cannot be auxiliary respiratory musculature anymore, a strong development of the respiratory muscles becomes necessary. Without a great increase of muscle volume this is accomplished by the more efficient angle of insertion at the processus uncinati.

Zimmer (1935) during his registrations of wing and trunk motions, observes an outward motion of the superior coracoid during downstroke and the opposite motion during upstroke of the wings. He suggests that these motions of the coracoids have effects on the thorax and could modify the respiratory motions. However, it is shown that the superior coracoid and the anterior scapula are separated from the anterior part of the rib cage, on which they are situated, by interposed diverticula of the cervical and interclavicular air sacs (Fig. 4a–c). These diverticula which substitute for each other are found in all flying species, very marked in long and well flying birds like pigeons, buzzards, gulls, ducks and song birds, but also in penguins. The cushion of these air sacs consequently saves the thorax from the effects of the wing motions.

But also indirectly, because of the various fillings of these air sacs, the respiration is hardly affected, for the axillary diverticula of the interclavicular air sac are well developed under the shoulder joint, between the muscle insertions in all well flying species. Now if the axillary diverticula are compressed during the downstroke of the wing, the diverticulum between coracoid and scapula and the anterior ribs is expanded during the outward motion of the shoulder joint; all that happens is a displacement of the air within the interclavicular air sac. The cervical air sac, if it is participating in the development of diverticula to a greater extent, may also experience variations in volume to a lesser degree. The specialization of the locomotor system of birds results in an independence of the systems for motions of the wings and legs from the system for the trunk, so that they cannot influence the respiratory motions.

Thus the old question of the relation between wing and respiratory motions is basically clarified. Because of the difficulty of the investigation only a few observations on this problem are existent as yet. Zimmer (1935) observed a synchronization between downstroke and inspiration and between upstroke and expiration in pigeons and crows; however, he suggests that this synchronization is not necessarily resulting from the construction of the locomotor system. Fraenkel (1934) reports to have demonstrated 4–5 respiratory motions per second and 15–20 wing strokes in the same time interval in the chaffinch, in the pigeon on the contrary he observed synchronization of respiratory and wing motions. Synchronization is also shown in the pigeon by Tomlinson and McKinnon (1957). Lord, Bellrose, and Cochran (1962) could very conclusively demonstrate that in the northern mallard one respiratory motion was accompanied by 2 wing strokes, and Tomlinson (1963) showed that in a gull species, a northern mallard, a pintail and a lesser scamp 3.5 to 7.3 wing strokes were performed per one inspiration, the larger the animal, the slower was its respiration and the more wing strokes were counted per breath. Tucker (1968a) reported for the budgerigar according to the corresponding flight velocity at a constant frequency of 840 wing strokes/min a respiratory frequency of 199 to 270 breaths/min. Berger, Roy, and Hart (1970) showed in 10 species, "that respiration of birds in flight is usually co-ordinated with wing beats but the co-ordination is not obligatory. Respiration synchronous with wing beats (1:1 co-ordination) was found only in pigeons and crows. Quails, ducks and pheasants, birds with relatively high wing beat frequencies showed a 5:1 co-ordination. Other species exhibited one of 10 other types of co-ordination, and even during flight the type of co-ordination changed."

These data confirm the conclusions, drawn from the construction, of an independence between respiratory and wing motions. In some species steadily, in others occasionally, a synchronization will be found. Size of the bird, type of flight and momentary performance are usually responsible for the fixation of inspirational frequency and sequence of wing beats. Tucker (1968a) has formulated a relation between respiratory and wing beat frequency according to the body weight, using and combining data of the body weight-oxygen consumption-relation (Lasiewski and Dawson, 1967) and of the body weight-wing beat frequency-relation (Greenewalt, 1962). This relation postulated that birds of the size of pigeons have an identical inspiratory and wing beat frequency determined by body weight, while larger birds breathe faster than they move their wings, and species smaller than pigeons exhibit a lesser frequency of inspiration than of wing beats. If both motions are performed with approximately the same velocity, a synchronization becomes meaningful. The presence of rhythmic accompanying motions without a mechanical coupling is well known from the human locomotor system.

Paleopulmo and Neopulmo — Two Structurally Different Parts of the Avian Lung

The dorsolateral surface of the lung exhibits very different features in the various species of birds. In a song bird, a pigeon or a chicken the surface is regularly occupied by closely adjoining parabronchi (Fig. 25b, c). In injection casts often the superficial subdivision of the parabronchial lumina into atria is recognized (Fig. 25b). Many other species, ducks, swans and gulls, owls, buzzards and parrots show the series of dorsobronchi, namely their dorsal portions, at the dorsal and cranial half of the dorsolateral lung surface (Figs. 23c, 25a). In cranes, cormorants and auks the dorsobronchi are superficially spread out in their whole course (Fig. 23a, b), and in storks, emus and penguins not only the dorsobronchi are situated at the surface all together, but the primary bronchus, coming from the lung hilus, reaches the surface directly and then turns towards caudal and, passing at the surface, opens into its ostium of the abdominal air sac (Figs. 20a, 23a).

In penguins the primary bronchus passes in the margin between the lateral thoracic wall and the horizontal septum towards the ostium at the caudal lung margin. During its course it gives off the dorsobronchi towards dorsal (Fig. 20a). Directly after the entrance of the primary bronchus into the lung hilus, the ventrobronchi arise (Figs. 28a, 32a). Between these two layers of secondary bronchi the tube system of the parabronchi is stretched out. The compact mass of the parabronchi, functioning in respiration, together with its vessels is enclosed between the two layers of secondary bronchi as in a sandwich (Fig. 32a). In penguins this sandwich occupies the whole lung. The great laterobronchus is very short and leads into the posterior thoracic air sac which is situated directly beneath the primary bronchus and the horizontal septum. The other small laterobronchus turns towards ventral and directs its parabronchi, likewise as the dorsobronchi, towards the ventrobronchi (Figs. 20a–c, 28a, 32a).

This structure which is so clearly demonstrated in the penguin lung, is repeated in the lungs of all other birds. Thus the ramifications of the ventrobronchi from the primary bronchus, directly after its entrance into the lung hilus, with their acute angle, specifically directed towards cranial, is a very constant feature; also, their extension on the whole ventral surface of the lung with their characteristic ramification and distribution, including the connections to the cervical, interclavicular and anterior thoracic air sacs (Figs. 28b, 29a–c, 32b, c, 33a–c). Constant is also the ramification and course of the dorsobronchi which originate from the primary bronchus behind the vestibulum as soon as it has turned caudally. Their ramification and distribution in the dorsolateral lung surface is also completely regular and characteristic to the dorsobronchi (Figs. 24a–c, 26a–c, 32b, c, 33a–c). As in penguin lungs, the stretched network of the parabronchi together with the vascular tree of the lung is also enclosed between dorsobronchi and ventrobronchi. This sandwich of the avian lung, with primary bronchus, ventrobronchi and dorsobronchi, compact mass of the parabronchi and vascular tree is named "paleopulmo" in the following discussion.

The paleopulmo is characterized by the high regularity of the structure and arrangement of all individual parts. This paleopulmo represents the whole lung in penguins, while in all other birds it constitutes the largest part of the lung, with 80% or more of the parabronchial volume. The paleopulmo may then be demonstrated very easily in all avian lungs. Only in its caudolateral portion it is covered by a newly developing network of parabronchi. Dorsally and cranially the superficial layer of the dorsobronchial terminal ramifications will always be recognized, even if partly provided with respiratory tissue. The anterior margin of the dorsolateral surface of the lung is always formed by the terminals of the anterior ventrobronchi which have curved around the margin from ventral. The ventrobronchi always also form the ventral surface of the lung except the posterior ventrolateral marginal zone. Those laterobronchi which do not communicate with the posterior thoracic air sac, give off parabronchi into the interior of the lung, in the direction towards the ventrobronchi. The vascular tree also can be found in corresponding arrangement and distribution in all lungs.

Vos (1937), in his report of the lack of "recurrent bronchi" in penguins, states that the caudolateral part of the penguin lung is only "poorly developed". This is true; for penguins lack the network of parabronchi which is found in most birds between primary and laterobronchus and posterior air sacs. The development of this network may be pursued via a whole series of intermediary types. In storks and emus a few parabronchi arise from the posterior primary bronchus, at its side directed towards ventrolateral, cross link and terminate laterally in the funnel-shaped ostia of the primary and laterobronchus into the posterior air sacs (Fig. 32b). In cranes, cormorants and auks this network of parabronchi is a little more expanded already (Figs. 23a, b, 24a, b). It originates not only from the primary bronchus, but also from the laterobronchi and, condensed into saccobronchi already, terminates laterally in the large ostia of the primary and laterobronchus into the posterior air sacs. Because of the increase of this parabronchial network the primary bronchus is shifted towards dorsal from the inferior lateral lung margin (Figs. 24b, c, 26a, 32c).

In cranes these parabronchi originate already from the whole external surface of the primary bronchus, beginning at the point where it turns towards caudal (Fig. 24b). Thereby the primary bronchus does not reach the lateral lung surface anymore. With the further development of this parabronchial net, the primary bronchus is not only shifted towards dorsal but also far into the lung interior.

Thus this new parabronchial net arises from the dorsobronchi, too, so that the latter also are displaced from the lung surface, as in ducks, swans, gulls, owls, buzzards and parrots (Figs. 26a, 32c, 33a, 34b). If this process of parabronchial expansion is very marked and if the smaller branches of the dorsobronchi at the same time have a parabronchial wall structure, larger bronchi cannot be distinguished anymore at the dorsolateral lung surface; parabronchi determine the construction of this lung portion, as in song birds, pigeons and chickens (Figs. 26b, c, 33b, c, 34c).

This parabronchial net which provides an additional communication between the primary bronchus and the laterobronchi and the posterior air sacs is termed "neopulmo" in the following discussion (Fig. 34b, c). It is developed and grows in volume in the course of the phylogenetic development of the birds. However, even if the neopulmo is maximally developed, the origins of its parabronchi never extend beyond that cranial point, where the primary bronchus turns towards caudal and gives rise to the first dorsobronchus. Besides from the primary bronchus, the neopulmonal parabronchi may also arise from the proximal parts of the dorsobronchi, even from that branch of the first dorsobronchus that runs towards lateroventral in order to supply the part of the anterior lung lying beneath the primary bronchus which is displaced upwards. Additionally, the parabronchi of the neopulmo arise from the laterobronchi which direct their paleopulmonal parabronchi towards medial. Besides, they often originate from the large latero-bronchus connecting the posterior thoracic air sac. The parabronchial net of the neopulmo is then aligned towards the ostia of the primary and the large latero-bronchus, in the funnel-shaped lateral parts of which they terminate (Fig. 31). Often, the parabronchi are condensed into saccobronchi shortly before their lateral termination in these two ostia, more seldom, as in plovers, curlews and sandpipers and in song birds into a longer saccobronchus into the abdominal air sac (Figs. 23c, 24c, 25a, c, 26a, c, 32b, 33a).

With the increasing development of a neopulmonal network as an additional connection between primary bronchus and air sacs, the diameter of the primary bronchus decreases markedly in its posterior portion. This process has progressed farthest in song birds in which the last portion of the primary bronchus is reduced to parabronchial width (Figs. 26c, 33c). Functionally, their abdominal air sac is completely connected via the neopulmo.

The connection of the posterior thoracic air sac is developed differently. At first the neopulmo terminates laterally in the funnel-shaped ostia of the latero-bronchus via more or less marked saccobronchi; the laterobronchus becomes continually narrower in relation to the arising parabronchi. However, the latero-bronchus always remains as a very wide communication with the primary bron-chus. In particular species, for instance the loons, the splitting of the lateral ostium of the neopulmo from that of the laterobronchus is initiated. This splitting has been completed in song birds. In these species the laterobronchial opening is situated more in the middle of the inferior lung surface (Figs. 15, 29c), and there marks the border between paleopulmo and neopulmo which occupies the caudolateral part of the lung. The ostia of the neopulmo lie at the lung margin (Figs. 24a–c, 26a–c, 28b, 29a–c) however, they may have a larger ostial zone.

In the highly developed neopulmo that is found in gulls, ducks and swans, the parabronchi of the neopulmo arise from the primary bronchus, the laterobronchi and the initial portions of the dorsobronchi. Cranially they also originate from the first branch of the dorsobronchus which runs directly towards ventral (Figs. 25a, 26a, 30a, 34b). In a higher type of the neopulmo, as it is found in plovers, curlews and sandpipers and most markedly in fowllike and song birds, this cranial origin from the first dorsobronchial branch is taken over by the lateral branch of the first ventrobronchus (Figs. 25b, c, 26b, c, 34c). Then the first branch of the first dorsobronchus, running towards ventral, obliterates, and the neopulmo occupies the whole lateroventral part of the lung. Thus, not only that part of the parabronchi arising from the lateral branch of the first ventrobronchus but also that from the lateral branch of the second ventro-bronchus is connected to the neopulmo. Thereby this part of the lung, lying wholly laterally and ventrally which originally belonged to the paleopulmo, is now arranged into the neopulmo.

The neopulmo differs from the paleopulmo also in that it shows considerable variations in the development of saccobronchi, both from species to species and partly within the same species. Great individual variations are also found in the small new laterobronchi which are additionally developed in the parabronchial net of the neopulmo of large species (Fig. 30a, b). They represent a connection between primary bronchus and parabronchial net and often are not wider than parabronchi, but characterized by very numerous parabronchial ramifications at their walls. They do not only vary in position, number and size, but they also lie in the midst of the parabronchial net of the neopulmo. The branches of the paleopulmonal vascular tree, ramifying in front of and under the primary bronchus, pass through the neopulmo accompanying the parabronchial net. Thereby they differ from the vessels of the paleopulmo. Within a particular species, however, the size of the neopulmo is very constant, independent of the observable variety of its construction. The neopulmo never exceeds about 20% of the lung volume, and usually, even if it is well developed, occupies about 10% of the parabronchial mass of the whole lung.

It may be summarized that a paleopulmo is present in all birds; it follows a fixed, invariable type of construction, the sandwich construction with primary bronchus, the two superficial layers of ventrobronchi and dorsobronchi and the compact mass of the parallel, cross linked parabronchi. The paleopulmo is exclusively existent in penguins. In all other birds, beginning very small in storks and emus a neopulmo is added which places itself externally on the primary bronchus, the dorsobronchi and laterobronchi, at the same time originating from them. The neopulmo is developed as an accessory parabronchial network connecting the posterior air sacs with the primary bronchus. If it is well developed, never exceeding 20% of the total lung volume, however, the neopulmo displaces the primary bronchus towards dorsal and deep into the interior of the lung, occupying the caudolateral part of the lung. It terminates either in the lateral portions of the funnel-shaped ostia of the primary and laterobronchus into the posterior air sacs or with saccobronchi of its own which are separated from the ostia of the large bronchi. The neopulmo is separated from the paleopulmo by the primary bronchus as well as by the dorsobronchi and laterobronchi; however, parabronchial communications exist between neopulmo and paleopulmo passing in between these bronchi. If the neopulmo extends so far cranially that the latero-ventral branch of the first dorsobronchus is reduced and the neopulmo joins the parabronchial net of the lateral branches of the first and second ventro-bronchi, a wide communication between the parabronchial systems of the neo-pulmo and paleopulmo originates in this lateroventral part of the lung.

In this type of the neopulmo which has reached its highest development, as in plovers, curlews and sandpipers, fowllike and song birds, its parabronchial net is not only directly connected to the ostia into the abdominal and posterior thoracic air sacs which may even be separate, as in song birds, but the neo-pulmo indeed has received a direct connection to the accessory lateral ostia into the anterior thoracic and interclavicular air sacs via its connection to the parabronchial net of the lateral branches of the first and second ventrobronchus. Thus special relations are resulting for the air sac connections of the highly developed neopulmo.

The Ventilation of the Paleopulmo and its Flow Dynamic Regulation According to Hazelhoff

The development of air capillaries, the resulting immobility of the lung, the lack of a blindly terminating bronchial tree and the connection of the bronchial system to the large air sacs require a type of respiration different from that known in mammals. This has most resolutely been advocated by Hazelhoff (1943, 1951); therefore the following considerations base on his work. Basing on Dotterweich (1936), Hazelhoff states a theory of flow dynamic regulation of the air through the paleopulmo during inspiration and expiration, using his good anatomical knowledge and the results of his physiological experiments. All ana-tomical structures important for Hazelhoff's theory are demonstrated in this study as constant structural elements of the paleopulmo of birds, especially those diameters and angles of ramification which are supposed to be responsible for the regulation of the air flow. Among them the following are significant: origin of the ventrobronchi with rigidly extended openings and alignment of their initial portions towards cranial, forming an acute angle with the primary bronchus, then following a variously wide dilatation of the ventrobronchi; origin of the dorsobronchi from the convexity of the posterior primary bronchus which runs at the lateral lung surface or beneath it towards caudal, with an alignment of the narrow initial portions of the dorsobronchi which can be regulated in their diameter, towards cranial forming an acute angle with the primary bronchus; origin of the one or few laterobronchi opposite to the anterior dorsobronchi, their initial portions also forming an acute angle towards cranial with the primary bronchus; connection of the ventilating posterior air sacs to the primary and large laterobronchus (Fig. 39). In the following discussion, using this general outline of the paleopulmonal construction, it is attempted to understand Hazel-hoff's theory also by the differences in pressure occurring in the bronchial system and to discuss some of the functional consequences.

During the inspiratory phase the posterior air sacs are expanded to a very large extent (Fig. 39a). Resulting from the difference in pressure between sur-rounding air and the interior of the posterior air sacs a strong flow of air enters the posterior air sacs through the primary and laterobronchus. In the anterior portion of the primary bronchus with the branchings of the ventrobronchi

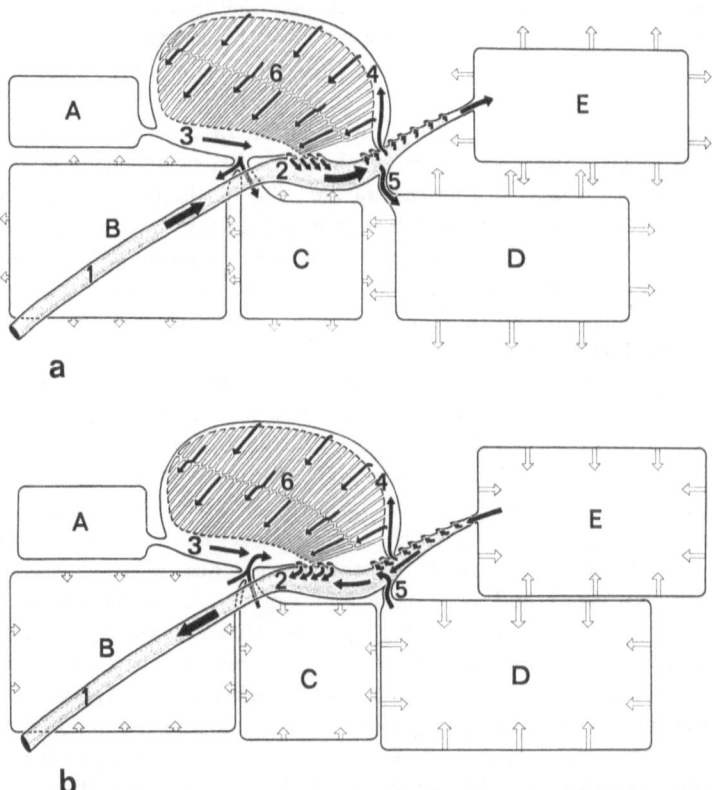

Fig. 39a and b. Scheme of the paleopulmo and the connections of the large air sacs. The whole bronchial system of the paleopulmo is connected parallel to the air passage through the primary bronchus into the posterior air sacs and back. The estimated way of the air through the paleopulmo according to Hazelhoff has been drawn with black arrows. a) Inspiratory phase. b) Expiratory phase. The length of the white arrows expresses the estimated amount of air sac dilatation or compression, the thickness of the black arrows the estimated intensity of the air flow in the particular parts of the bronchial system. The air flows in the same direction through the paleopulmo during both respiratory phases, only in the primary bronchus and in the laterobronchus the direction of air flow is changed corresponding to the respiratory phases.—A cervical, B interclavicular, C anterior thoracic, D posterior thoracic, E abdominal air sac. 1 trachea, 2 primary bronchus, 3 ventrobronchi, 4 dorsobronchi, 5 laterobronchi, 6 parabronchial net between dorsobronchi and ventrobronchi

directed cranially, as far as the end of the vestibulum, a strong but still laminar flow originates. The air flow is divided at the origin of the large laterobronchus and then passes through it into the posterior thoracic air sac and through the posterior primary bronchus into the abdominal air sac. — Hazelhoff studied a suspension of particles in either water or air in artificially ventilated dead birds through the thin dorsobronchial wall. He observed a constant flow out of the primary bronchus into the dorsobronchi in the inspiratory phase. He was able to make the same observations on glass models.

According to Hazelhoff's theory, the inspiratory flow in the primary bronchus must feed an air flow into the dorsobronchi and back into the primary bronchus via the parabronchi and ventrobronchi (Fig. 39a). Hazelhoff explains the direction of this flow by the flow dynamic characteristics of the specific portions of the bronchial system. The angle of ramification of the ventrobronchi, directed towards cranial, is supposed to produce those conditions which allow the pumping off of air through them during inspiration. The position of the dorsobronchial openings on the convex side of the posterior primary bronchus probably is responsible for the inflow of air into the dorsobronchi during the same inspiratory phase. The origin of the opposite large laterobronchus initially, directed towards cranial, into the posterior thoracic air sac also positively influences the inflow into the dorsobronchi (Fig. 39a).

A number of other structural characteristics which are constantly observed, are significant for the understanding of the concept of air flow. The ventrobronchi dilate very markedly after their origin from the primary bronchus, usually up to 3–8 times their initial cross sectional area. The dorsobronchi also dilate shortly after their origin, however, never as markedly as the ventrobronchi. Besides, the primary bronchus, along with the ramification of the ventrobronchi towards caudal, increases in diameter, to become continually narrower in the course of the dorsobronchial and laterobronchial origins. If the neopulmo is highly developed, the primary bronchus in its posterior portion shortly after the origin of the last dorsobronchus may functionally be completely substituted by the neopulmonal parabronchial net for the connection of the abdominal air sac. The laterobronchus into the posterior thoracic air sac always remains as a wide connection to this air sac, even if the neopulmo is well developed (Fig. 40). The anterior air sacs which are hardly or not at all ventilated, are always connected to ventrobronchi, near their origins and have accessory ostia from the lateral parabronchial net. These accessory ostia receive connections to the neopulmonal parabronchial net, if a neopulmo is highly developed.

If the pressures which are generated in the particular portions of the bronchial system during strong inspiration, are considered at first, following hypothesis may be stated: The same lowering of the air pressure is effective in the primary bronchus and the air sacs. Thereby a difference in pressure is generated from the ventrobronchi to the primary bronchus. Corresponding relations should be true for the dorsobronchi. However, considering the much larger total cross sectional area of the ventrobronchi compared to the dorsobronchi, a difference in pressure could be produced between these two groups of bronchi which could lead to a current of air from the dorsobronchi via the parabronchi to the ventrobronchi. Of importance could also be the relation of cross sectional area at the origin to maximal cross sectional area which is different for dorsobronchi and ventrobronchi. These conditions indicate that the initial portion of the dorsobronchi must exhibit a higher pressure than the ventrobronchi during inspiration, consequently a lesser decrease in pressure in the whole system. Considering the pressure proportions a lesser reduction of pressure must then exist in the posterior primary bronchus in order to render possible an inflow of air into the dorsobronchi. Perhaps this is caused by the continual decrease of the diameter of the primary bronchus along the dorsobronchial origins.

However, considering Hazelhoff's theory, perhaps a certain stagnation pressure appears at the origin of the dorsobronchi, due to the complicated flow dynamic conditions in the posterior primary bronchus which changes the pressure in such a manner as to facilitate the inflow into the dorsobronchi. These pressures must be maintained continually during inspiration by the inflow of air into the posterior air sacs which steadily expand. According to this hypothesis, the paleopulmo is continually perfused by the very complicated inspiratory flow in the primary bronchus causing a difference in pressure between dorsobronchi and ventrobronchi. This means that air from the paleopulmo is additionally transported along with the inspiratory air between the origins of the ventrobronchi and the dorsobronchi. Air circulates through the paleopulmo which is added to the flow through the primary bronchus at the ventrobronchial openings and at the same time expelled at the origin of the dorsobronchi (Fig. 39 a).

The synchronous action of all air sacs is unanimously advocated in the literature (Baer, 1896; Soum, 1896; Francois-Franck, 1906; Victorow, 1909; Scharnke, 1934), but only basing on qualitative studies. Measurements of pressure values are existent for only the trachea and the abdominal air sacs of the pigeon, as yet (Beerens, 1932). Therefore the pressure values in the different air sacs and in the various parts of the primary bronchus can only be estimated. If the primary inspiratory drop of pressure would be equal in all air sacs, the different size, the different length and the various diameters of the connections of the air sacs could cause not only different inflow velocities but also a various lowering of the pressure in the individual parts of the primary bronchus.

The posterior thoracic air sac is always connected to the primary bronchus via a short, wide laterobronchus, while the abdominal air sac has very various connections to the caudal primary bronchus; often it is connected to the primary bronchus only via the neopulmo. Thereby a greater drop in pressure could appear in the anterior portion of the primary bronchus — in the region of origin of the ventrobronchi — than in the posterior, where the dorsobronchi originate. This could be another factor, together with the narrowing of the primary bronchus, for the difference in pressure between dorsobronchi and ventrobronchi, necessary for a perfusion of the paleopulmo during inspiration. Not only the different cross sectional areas of the dorsobronchi and ventrobronchi, but also the points of origin which are specific to both groups of secondary bronchi and maintained constantly throughout all species of birds should have their functional significance.

It must be emphasized, however, that bronchial diameter and air sac size are specific to the individual groups of species and are subject to considerable variations from family to family (Figs. 1, 2, 5a–c, 6a–c, 23a–c, 24a–c, 25a–c, 26a–c, 28a, b, 29a–c, 32a–c, 33a–c). The pressure and perfusion relations will only be clarified by quantitative studies basing on the size relations or by measurements of the pressure at various points of the bronchial and air sac system in particular species. However, only by a comparison of different species a satisfactory explanation of the fundamental principles of function of the lung air sac system will be obtained, or it will be found that different types of function have been developed which find their anatomical expression in the different, considerably varying sizes of air sacs and bronchi.

Further anatomical facts must be considered in this discussion which advocate Hazelhoff's theory of air flow during the inspiratory phase. In the course of the origin of the ventrobronchi the cross sectional area of the primary bronchus increases about 20–50% in the different species, and then passes on as far as its bend towards caudal, with unchanged cross section. Starting there it gives rise to the dorsobronchi and laterobronchi and becomes narrower corresponding to the cross section of the bronchi branched off. If the inspiratory flow receives inflow out of the ventrobronchi — according to Hazelhoff — the flow velocity could remain constant for identical intensity of flow because of the increase of the cross sectional area of the primary bronchus. The corresponding could occur in the posterior primary bronchus because of the origins of the dorsobronchi and laterobronchi.

In all birds only the thin dividing membranes of the ventrobronchial openings into the primary bronchus are stiffened by embedded cartilage. Thus, if the pressure in the primary bronchus is lowered to a higher degree, a collapse of the openings may be prevented and the air may flow unrestrained out of the ventrobronchi. Dorsobronchi and laterobronchi do not possess such a support of their openings into the primary bronchus and, if they are to fit into this concept, do not need it. On the contrary, using their musculature they have the possibility of regulating their cross section and thereby the inflow of air.

The anterior air sacs which always have a wide communication with the ventrobronchi, experience only a slight dilatation during inspiration. Only the anterior thoracic air sac, if it is extended further caudally, may expand more markedly. The drop in pressure of these air sacs would effect the ventrobronchi and thus amplify a flow out of the parabronchi from the dorsobronchi or even generate it. The type of connection of the anterior air sacs underlines these functional concepts explicitly.

During the expiratory phase a pressure increase is generated in the posterior air sacs which leads to a flow through the primary bronchus and the trachea. The expiratory flow in the posterior primary bronchus is directed straightly towards the openings of the medial and anterior dorsobronchi, while the flow out of the large laterobronchus (and therefore out of the posterior thoracic air sac) is directed towards the opposite dorsobronchial openings because of its angle of ramification from the primary bronchus. Thus a considerable portion of the expiratory flow is directed into the dorsobronchial openings. Another part flows out through the vestibulum, uniting with the outflow out of the ventrobronchi, and is ejected via the trachea. The expiratory flow out of the ventrobronchi is consisting of the air coming from the dorsobronchi via the parabronchi and the air from the anterior air sacs which are slightly compressed (Fig. 39b).

Considering the probable pressure relations, the perfusion of the paleopulmo during the expiratory phase is easier to understand. The increase in pressure in the posterior air sacs shows also effects in the primary bronchus and continues into the dorsobronchi. For the air flow, generated by the increase in pressure in the primary bronchus, is directed on the openings of the dorsobronchi in such a manner that it may continue unrestrained into the dorsobronchi. The alignment of the dorsobronchial initial portions towards cranial is the decisive basis for this effect. Thereby the expiratory flow is divided in one through the paleopulmo and another partial flow through the vestibulum into the anterior primary bronchus. At the origin of the ventrobronchi both flows unite again. Considering the increase of the cross section of the primary bronchus and the division of the air flow it can be seen that both factors cause a decrease in pressure towards the anterior primary bronchus. Thus, the difference in pressure between dorsobronchi and ventrobronchi is guaranteed which maintains the perfusion of the paleopulmo. Here also, the larger cross section of the ventrobronchi is of a certain importance, since it reduces the flow resistance. These relations are probably not disturbed by the slight inflow of expiratory air out of the anterior air sacs, since the difference in pressure between dorsobronchi and ventrobronchi may be great enough.

Summarizing, the following may be stated: the anterior portion of the primary bronchus with its ventrobronchi originating directly behind each other and being directed towards cranial in their initial portions, and with its dilatation, the vestibulum, represents that structure which probably pumps off air out of the ventrobronchi, with the help of a drop in pressure, during the inflow of the inspiratory air into the posterior air sacs. The posterior portion of the primary bronchus with the originating dorsobronchi and laterobronchi is that part of the bronchial system which receives the air that has been pressed out of the posterior air sacs during the expiratory phase, into the dorsobronchi directed towards cranial. In both respiratory phases the dorsobronchi would be the place in the paleopulmo which shows the highest pressure — according to this concept — because of the specific arrangement and structure of the secondary bronchi. Thereby, in both respiratory phases a flow of respiratory air from the dorsobronchi into the ventrobronchi via the parabronchi would be generated, a concept that is underlined by the always larger cross section of the ventrobronchi. Another argument for these relations is that the dorsobronchi which must always show a higher pressure compared to the ventrobronchi, never have any air sac connections. This may be an important anatomical requirement for an unimpaired functioning of the pressure and flow relations.

An exact consideration of the construction of the bronchial system and of the functional hypotheses, basing on it, advocates an unidirectional perfusion of the lung, independent of the respiratory phases, as has been postulated by Hazelhoff. Even though the avian lung is mostly a system of rigid tubes, the expiration is not simply an inversion of inspiration. If it was an inversion, all pressure and flow relations would also have to be inversed and the respiratory air would be directed exactly inverse (Scheid, personal communication), an unidirectional perfusion, independent of the respiratory phases, could therefore not exist. Now, during inspiration a drop in pressure exists in the anterior primary bronchus, causing a suction of air out of the paleopulmo, while during expiration an increase in pressure appears in the posterior primary bronchus which is lowered in the anterior primary bronchus. It is suggested that the specific arrangement and opening of the ventrobronchi and dorsobronchi must lead to the unidirectional perfusion of the paleopulmo under these pressure conditions, principally varying with the respiratory phases.

This type of construction of the paleopulmo fundamentally present in all birds, is not changed even if the neopulmo is highly developed (Fig. 41). Then, the primary bronchus in its function of connecting the abdominal air sac, is substituted by the neopulmonal parabronchial net, a fact that has no influence on the flow in the region of dorsobronchial origin. The parabronchi of the neopulmo originating from the initial portions of the dorsobronchi, too, support the flow into the dorsobronchi during inspiration, likewise during expiration (Fig. 41). Only in the anterior lateral portion of the lung, if the parabronchial network of a highly developed neopulmo communicates through the lateral branches of the first and second ventrobronchus (Fig. 34c), the conditions for a perfusion during the inspiratory phase are not completely understood as yet; during expiration air flows out of the air sacs via the neopulmonal parabronchi into the lateral ventrobronchial branches and the primary bronchus. It seems to be significant that at least quite a number of those species which have a highly developed neopulmo, at the same time have a large anterior thoracic air sac, as in plovers, curlews, sandpipers and fowllike birds. This air sac is connected with its accessory ostium via this lateral parabronchial net and possible the common development of the laterocranial neopulmo and a large anterior thoracic air sac has a functional significance.

An unidirectional air flow through the paleopulmo has been postulated before Dotterweich (1936) and Hazelhoff (1943, 1951) already by Brandes (1924), Bethe (1925), Portier (1928), Dotterweich (1930a, 1933) and Vos (1935). However, they tried to explain this air flow by valves which have never been demonstrated. Besides Hazelhoff's theory and the considerations basing on the anatomical structures which have been presented in this study, a number of further observations advocate an unidirectional air flow: Dotterweich (1930b) and Vos (1935) studied natural deposits of soot (pigeons living in railway stations) and deposits artificially induced by inhalation of soot. They found that the soot is present in the posterior portion of the primary bronchus, the large laterobronchus, the initial portions of the dorsobronchi and the parabronchial net between primary bronchus and posterior air sacs in larger amounts; it is accumulated in the posterior thoracic and abdominal air sacs. Very little soot only could generally be found in the ventrobronchi and the anterior air sacs. This is completely in accordance with the author's findings on some intensely sooted city birds. Such a distribution of the soot is only possible, however, if the inspiratory flow enters the parabronchi via the dorsobronchi; the postulated unidirectional air circulation must therefore exist. It must be mentioned that Walter (1934) could not confirm this type of experimental soot absorption. Perhaps this could have occurred because he forced his pigeons to pant, due to overheating the birds during the experiment, or because the birds suffered from hypoxia during the tests.

Besides the arrangement, width and angle relations of the bronchial system, explained in the foregoing discussion, a further anatomical finding advocates the unidirectional air flow. The ventrobronchial walls are never completely lined by respiratory tissue, at the most, small parts of such tissue can be found at the inside of the lung around the terminating parabronchi. On the contrary, in many avian species, most markedly developed in song and fowllike birds and pigeons, not only the small dorsobronchial branches, but even their large stems are completely surrounded by a mantle of respiratory tissue, that is as well developed as in the parabronchi. This and the absorption of soot advocates the concept that fresh inspiratory air always enters the dorsobronchi and not the ventrobronchi and that maximally used expiratory air always leaves through the ventrobronchi. However, these findings cannot confirm whether this happens only during the expiratory phase or also during inspiration.

Soum (1896), Dotterweich (1933), Plantefol and Scharnke (1934), Scharnke (1934), Makowski (1938a), Graham (1939), Zeuthen (1942), Shepard, Sladen, Peterson, and Enns (1959), and Piiper, Drees, and Scheid (1970) have analyzed the air out of the different air sacs. It could be shown that interclavicular and anterior thoracic air sacs always have a high CO_2-content, with an average of about 5%, and an O_2-content of 14–15%, while the posterior air sacs generally have a higher O_2-content and a lower CO_2-content, still markedly varying with the different respiratory phases. These findings advocate the unidirectional flow of the respiratory air through the paleopulmonal parabronchial system; for, in this concept of air circulation, only air that has already passed the parabronchi could reach the anterior air sacs. It must be considered, however, that the anterior air sacs have a large dead space in which the air can only be exchanged with difficulties, already for anatomical reasons.

The different participation of the various parts of the lung air sac system in the ventilation is also clearly expressed by the determination of the volume of the respiratory tract using the wash-out method (Scheid and Piiper, 1969) which demonstrated three differently ventilated compartments, the topographical correspondence of which is still not known as yet. That compartment that is exchanged in the least time is probably corresponding to the air volume of the bronchial system plus the paleopulmo, the following compartment that of the air volume of the posterior air sacs, while that part exchanged after the longest time interval must probably be sought in the anterior air sacs.

Now, if all previous data are summarized, it is almost proved that a flow of respiratory air continual during inspiration and expiration, passes from the primary bronchus through the dorsobronchi and the parabronchial net and then back through the ventrobronchi. Such a circulation would be of a great functional significance, because then the dead space in the total bronchial system could be kept minimally small. This could be a decisive factor in the high functional efficiency of the avian lung, especially in well flying species.

First experimental evidence of an unidirectional flow through the paleopulmo according to Hazelhoff was recently given by Scheid and Piiper (1971) for the duck. With the use of devices measuring the flow in the second and third dorsobronchus they were able to show a continual flow during inspiration and expiration. However, a physical explanation cannot be given at the moment. Besides this principal proof of Hazelhoff's theory, the most remarkable fact of these findings is that the air flow in the dorsobronchi is not reduced to zero, when the flow in the primary bronchus is reversed from inspiration to expiration, but that it persists to quite an extent. Towards the end and after expiration which takes much longer time than the inspiration, the flow in the dorsobronchi approaches zero. By measurements during the thermoregulatory panting which showed relatively weaker intensities of flow in the dorsobronchi, the capability of regulating the paleopulmonal perfusion of the lung was qualitatively demonstrated at the same time.

In such an air circulation the flow of the inspiratory and expiratory air which is generated by the changes in volume and thus in pressure of the posterior air sacs, feeds the air flow through the rigid tube system of the paleopulmo which is connected parallel to the primary bronchus (Figs. 39, 41). It is unknown, as yet, to what percentage the respiratory air passes through the parabronchi and therefore participates in the gas exchange, and to what extent it only passes through the large bronchi into the posterior air sacs and back. Calculations which have been made by Zeuthen (1942) with the use of the CO_2-content of the posterior air sacs and of the expiratory air in chickens, indicated that one third to one half of the air inspired, reach the air sacs via the parabronchi during inspiration, while on to two thirds are expired through the parabronchi during expiration. Besides, for artificially opened posterior air sacs the air flow necessary to pervent a cyanosis is supposed to be greater during a perfusion in the direction from trachea into the air sac than vice versa (Salt and Zeuthen, 1960). However, these data do not consider the connection of the posterior air sacs by the parabronchial net of the neopulmo. They only state a concept of the total system, neopulmo plus paleopulmo, which at the moment cannot be differentiated according to its shares in the gas exchange. Furthermore, it has not been clarified whether this relation is changed during the transition from respiration at rest to respiration in flight.

Calculations which have been made for the budgerigar by Tucker (1968a), show that in this species the oxygen consumption at rest up to the maximal flight velocity is directly proportional to the ventilation volume. The oxygen consumption is 6.2 to 6.6% of the volume, a finding that is in very good accordance with data of Soum (1896), Dotterweich (1936), Scharnke (1938), Makowski (1938a, b), Graham (1939), and Piiper, Drees and Scheid (1970) which found 13–14% oxygen in the expiratory air of pigeons, chickens and ducks. Especially the data of Tucker (1968a) allow the assumption that the constant values of the expiratory air are mainly determined by the physiologically fixed partial pressures in the end-expired air of the parabronchi. This assumption indicates that the inspiratory air is optimally used, consequently that the largest part of the inspiratory air must flow through the parabronchial net. Thereby the avian respiratory apparatus would have reached the theoretical optimum.

Tucker's (1968a) findings, however, base on a calculation of the ventilation from the respiratory loss of water during which the temperature of the expiratory air has not been measured; therefore they are only minimal values of the ventilation. Considering findings of Schmidt-Nielsen, Hainsworth, and Murrish (1970) the temperature of the expiratory air is primarily dependent on the temperature of the environment especially in small birds so that the water content of the expiratory air is of only small importance for the value of ventilation. Thus an O_2-difference between inspiratory and expiratory air of 2.0–3.3% results according to data of Berger, Hart, and Roy (1970) for 3 species of resting and flying birds and of Berger (personal communication) for buzzing hummingbirds. This represents a basal value which also is not changed at rest according to Berger (personal communication). These values, obtained by modern methods, therefore invalidate the data found in the older literature at least for the species investigated. These findings also show that the clarification of the ventilatory relations of the paleopulmo, especially the question to which extent the air flows through the paleo-pulmonal parabronchi and to which extent only through primary and latero-bronchus into the posterior air sacs, still requires intensive experimental research.

These assumptions show that intensive experimental research is still required for the clarification of the ventilation in the paleopulmo. Additionally a numerical analysis of the flow dynamic relations in the different parts of this bronchial system for the various respiratory phases should be made in different species, basing on an exact measurement of diameters, length and angle of ramification of the particular parts of the bronchial system. Together with these experimental studies perhaps the problem of the extent of a paleopulmonal regulation and control of the air flow by flow dynamic principles, and by the muscles in the primary and the laterobronchus, the initial portions of the dorsobronchi and the parabronchi, may be solved.

The Ventilation of the Neopulmo and the Problem of Respiration at Rest

As has been described, the connection of the posterior air sacs shows marked variations in the different avian species. In penguins it is connected to wide bronchi only (Fig. 39), in all other birds an increasing network of parabronchi between primary bronchus and laterobronchus and the air sacs is added (Fig. 40). The neopulmo does not influence the ventilation within the paleopulmo no matter how it is controlled (Fig. 41). An air sac connection through wide lumina is substituted by a number of narrow connections. If the total cross sectional area is not decreased, the flow velocity in the posterior primary bronchus seems also not to be altered. It must be considered, however, that the smaller lumina re-present a far greater flow resistance and therefore must have developed a larger total cross section in order to maintain the same flow intensity.

It is characteristic that the parabronchi never originate from the primary bronchus *before* its bend towards caudal. The connection to the posterior thoracic air sac is always made by a large laterobronchus, besides the connection through the neopulmo, even when the primary bronchus is wholly substituted by the neopulmo, as in song birds. The unimpaired ventilation of the paleopulmo is maintained even if the neopulmonal parabronchi arise from the initial portion of the dorsobronchi, since thereby the direction of the air flow is not altered in the dorsobronchi (Fig. 41).

The neopulmo does not influence the ventilation of the paleopulmo. However, if it reaches a certain size, it represents a new physiological factor. According to the width of the connecting laterobronchus and primary bronchus, a more or less great part of the respiratory air must perfuse the neopulmo on its way to and from the posterior air sacs during both inspiration and expiration (Fig. 40). This air flow is not only divided physiologically into many partial currents by the neopulmonal network but also participates in the gas exchange; for the neopulmo is formed by normally developed parabronchi which do not differ in structure from the paleopulmonal parabronchi.

In its function the network of the neopulmo shows a significant difference to the paleopulmo; for it necessarily is perfused in changing direction during inspiration and expiration (Fig. 40). Therefore the term "bronchi recurrentes"

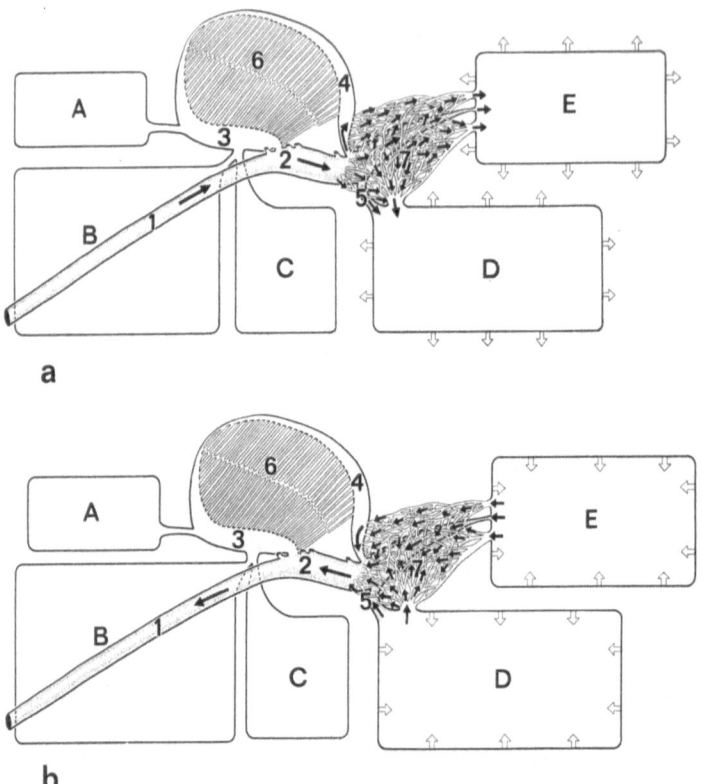

Fig. 40a and b. Scheme of the paleopulmo and the neopulmo and the connections of the large air sacs. While the bronchial system of the paleopulmo remains parallel to the primary bronchus, the neopulmo develops directly interposed in the air passage out of the primary bronchus into the posterior air sacs. The estimated way of the air through a lung with paleo-pulmo and neopulmo, as it is assumed during respiration at rest with slight respiratory amplitude, has been drawn with black arrows. a) Inspiratory phase. b) Expiratory phase. The length of the white arrows expresses the estimated amount of air sac dilatation or com-pression, the thin black arrows express the direction of the weak air flow, changing with the respiratory phases in the neopulmo. The paleopulmo is not ventilated.—*A* cervical, *B* interclavicular, *C* anterior and *D* posterior thoracic, *E* abdominal air sac. *1* trachea, *2* pri-mary bronchus, *3* ventrobronchi, *4* dorsobronchi, *5* laterobronchi, *6* parabronchial net between dorsobronchi and ventrobronchi, *7* accessory parabronchial net of the neopulmo between primary bronchus, laterobronchi and dorsobronchi and the posterior air sacs

of Schulze (1910) and Juillet (1911a, c, 1912b) for the saccobronchi is mis-leading. Thus it seems that only in the neopulmo the direction of flow that varies according to the respiratory phase is existent; this change in air flow had been postulated for the whole lung by many authors, for the last time by Salt and Zeuthen (1960).

Because of the interposition of the neopulmonal network between primary bronchus and posterior air sacs, a perfusion of the neopulmo with the inflowing and outflowing air takes place during the changes in volume of these posterior air sacs which is independent of the flow dynamic regulations. Always that amount of air flows through the neopulmo during inspiration and expiration which corresponds to their share of the total cross sectional area of the air sac connections. This share of the cross section can probably be regulated by the muscles both in the primary and large laterobronchus and the parabronchi. Especially in song birds, but also in pigeons and chickens the abdominal air sac is functionally completely, the posterior thoracic air sac to 50% connected via the neopulmo. In these species therefore the main portion of the respiratory air must pass the neopulmo during inspiration and expiration. This share is quite different in other species, according to the size of the neopulmo and the width of the large bronchi connecting the air sacs, until it is totally lacking in penguins which do not have a neopulmo.

Basing on these findings, the following hypothesis is stated: The flow dynamic regulation of the paleopulmonal ventilation requires certain minimal values of the flow velocity in the primary bronchus for its functioning, in order to generate sufficient differences in pressure which may overcome the flow resistance in its bronchial system. In the inspiratory phase, if this limiting value was undercut, the drop in pressure in the primary bronchus would not suffice to generate such a drop in pressure in the ventrobronchi which in turn generates a sufficiently great difference in pressure against the dorsobronchi that could supply the air flow through the parabronchi. The corresponding is true for the expiratory phase during which the increase in pressure in the dorsobronchi against the ventrobronchi has to be above that limiting value of the difference in pressure that allows the perfusion of the parabronchi.

Contrary to the paleopulmo, the neopulmo is perfused according to its share in the cross sectional area of the connections of the posterior air sacs, as soon as a change in pressure and thus an air flow is generated in the primary bronchus. This means that already at a minimal flow in the primary bronchus and that is at minimal difference in pressure which itself would not suffice to perfuse the paleopulmo, a gas exchange takes place in the neopulmo (Fig. 40). This is a situation occuring during respiration at rest. As soon as the bird in flight makes deeper respiratory excursions, the differences in pressure in the air sacs rise (Beerens, 1932; Scharnke, 1938) and at the same time the differences in pressure and consequently the flow velocity in the primary bronchus, establishing the basis necessary for a ventilation of the paleopulmo (Fig. 41).

Thereby, a differentiation in the development of the avian lung has been established in a smaller part — the neopulmo — for the respiration at rest and in a larger part — the paleopulmo — for the respiration during greater performance, in flight and during running. The neopulmo participates in the gas exchange during both respiratory stages. During respiration at rest it is capable of completely exchanging the small amount of respiratory air because of the small flow velocity, up to the physiological maximal value for the respiratory exchange, the end-parabronchial value (Scheid and Piiper, 1970). If the flow velocity in the neopulmo rises together with an increase of the respiratory volume, a quantitatively identical amount of gas is exchanged in the neopulmo, namely the volume of CO_2 and O_2 that can maximally be exchanged per unit time, but the larger amount of respiratory air in the same unit of the time is used relatively worse. In this case the necessary time of contact is not reached. Instead, a portion of this poorly exchanged air will flow through the paleopulmo where the gas exchange up to the end-parabronchial value may take place.

It is interesting in this connection that the metabolism and respiratory gas exchange of a bird increases during the transition from rest to flight: to the 10-fold (Berger, Hart, and Roy, 1970, for 3 larger species), the 11- to 14-fold (Tucker, 1969, for a gull), the 13- to 20-fold (Tucker, 1968a, 1969, for the budgerigar), up to the 25-fold of the value at rest (Zeuthen, 1942, for pigeons). An estimation of the size of the neopulmo shows that it occupies about 10% to maximally 20% of the total parabronchial mass. It follows that the neopulmo is well capable of performing the gas exchange at rest. The larger part of the lung, the paleopulmo, would then be used for the additional work which, however, in flight is a manyfold of the work at rest.

Therefore, most of the measurements of the gas content of the air sacs which have been performed at normal or slightly increased respiration at rest, must be evaluated from this point of view. In these experiments with chickens, pigeons and ducks (Soum, 1896; Dotterweich, 1933; Plantefol and Scharnke, 1934; Scharnke, 1934, 1938; Makowski, 1938a; Graham, 1939; Zeuthen, 1942; Shepard et al., 1959; Piiper, Drees, and Scheid, 1970) which all have a well developed neopulmo, therefore mainly the respiration and gas exchange through the neopulmo has been studied. Differences in the CO_2-content ranging from 1.29 to 5.15%, as Scharnke (1934) found in different measurements of air out of the abdominal air sac of the pigeon, could not be suited into a contemporary theory. In 1938 Scharnke found that a high CO_2-content is found in all posterior air sacs during respiration at rest which rapidly sinks during stronger respiration, while the O_2-content behaves vice versa. These and other data of the literature may be easily explained with the help of a detailed knowledge of the structure and the possible function of the paleopulmo and the neopulmo. Markedly varying values as those of Scharnke (1934, 1938) probably arise from the different participation of the paleopulmo in the gas exchange before the different measurements. However, the partly very considerable variations in the construction of the lung in the species studied must always be considered if the investigator wants to correctly interpret the values obtained.

Thus the old conflict between the concept of a direction of flow through the parabronchi changing synchronously with the respiratory phases (Soum, 1896; Scharnke, 1938; Zeuthen, 1942; Salt and Zeuthen, 1960) which actually occurs in the neopulmo, and the concept of an unidirectional perfusion during both inspiration and expiration (Brandes, 1924; Bethe, 1925; Vos, 1935; Dotterweich, 1936; Hazelhoff, 1943, 1951) that is very probably occurring in the paleopulmo, is solved (Fig. 41). This antagonism is more easily understandable because all experiments were performed on species of poultry which all have a well developed neopulmo.

Those families that have only a poorly developed neopulmo, as storks and emus or those as penguins in which it is totally lacking, display a different type of respiration. They have to carry out the respiration at rest with their paleopulmo, too. In penguins formations of crests in the posterior primary bronchus are found; these are directed towards the anterior dorsobronchi as

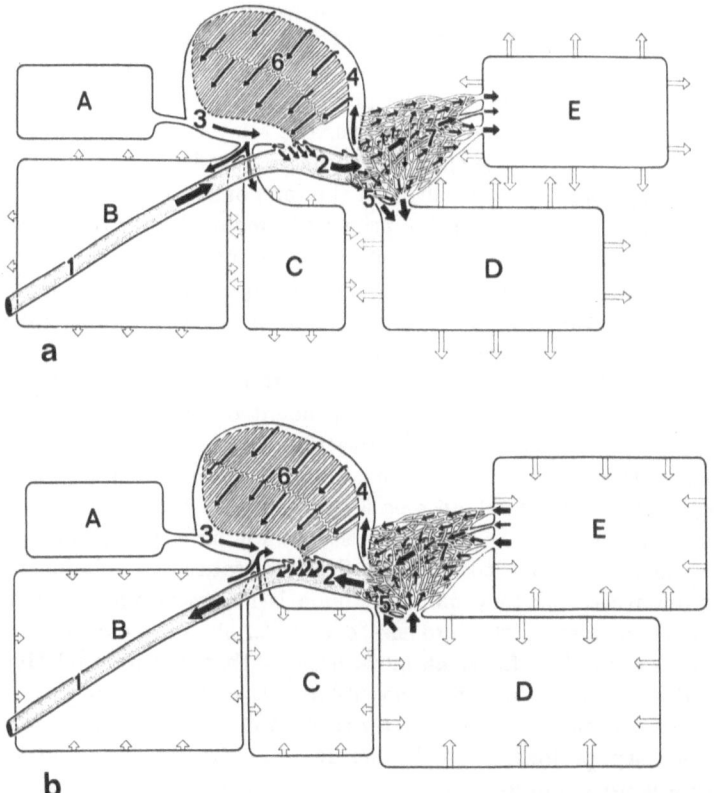

Fig. 41 a and b. Scheme of the air flow in a lung with paleopulmo and neopulmo, as it is assumed during respiration at maximum stress with great respiratory amplitude. a) Inspiratory phase. b) Expiratory phase. The length of the white arrows expresses the estimated amount of air sac dilatation or compression. The thickness of the black arrows expresses the estimated intensity of the air flow in the individual parts of the bronchial system. The neopulmo, correspondent to its connection, is perfused in changing directions during the respiratory phases, the paleopulmo is unidirectionally ventilated in both respiratory phases. *A* cervical, *B* interclavicular, *C* anterior and *D* posterior thoracic, *E* abdominal air sac. *1* trachea, *2* primary bronchus, *3* ventrobronchi, *4* dorsobronchi, *5* laterobronchi, *6* parabronchial net between dorsobronchi and ventrobronchi, *7* accessory parabronchial net of the neopulmo between primary bronchus, laterobronchi and dorsobronchi and the posterior air sacs

prolongation of the orifice of the laterobronchus which connects the posterior thoracic air sac. Possibly they have a significance in a better alignment of the expiratory flow into the dorsobronchi, especially for the respiration at rest. These crests are not found in other birds.

The families of penguins, storks and emus which have no or only a weakly developed neopulmo, are always represented only by large birds. Small species are lacking. Additionally these families have to be placed at the beginning of the phylogenetic system because of a number of features. All species standing systematically higher possess a neopulmo, even if only to a variable degree. In these, small species like most of the song birds, are also found. Thus the lung construction of the procellariids was of special interest for they are often systematically placed at the beginning of the natural system of birds; with storm petrel and leach's petrel they also have representatives of the small size of song birds. It was found that the procellariids also have a well developed neopulmo which resembles that of the gulls. The relations between lung structure and systematic position of the species need further studying.

The following conclusions result from the foregoing findings: the paleopulmo requires a minimal flow through the primary bronchus for its ventilation which is established by a certain minimal respiratory minute volume. In large birds, the air volume necessary to cover the oxygen requirement should be sufficient to establish the ventilation of the paleopulmo. If the bird size is considerably reduced, the respiratory minute volume necessary to cover the oxygen need sinks, together with its body volume, with the third power of the trunk length, or more exactly, since it is very much dependent on the surface, with a value of $^2/_3$ to $^3/_4$ of the third power. The cross sectional area of the bronchi, especially of the primary bronchus, which is responsible for the flow intensity for a given respiratory minute volume, as an area is lowered with the second power of the trunk length. Besides, it can be shown that small birds have relatively wider bronchi, probably in order to keep the flow resistance low. Consequently, an increasing relative respiratory minute volume is necessary for a ventilation of the paleopulmo at rest, if the bird size decreases. A lung, only developed as paleopulmo, is unefficient for small birds, because they require a relatively very high respiratory minute volume for the ventilation at rest. The neopulmo solves this problem since it is not tied to such a size relation in its function. Even very small species may perform a respiration at rest without additional work. At work the respiratory minute volume is always so great in small species that the paleopulmo can be ventilated. Consequently, it is imaginable that the neopulmo has been a necessary requirement for the phylogenetic development of the various small bird types which has made the class of birds so various and successful. This is in accordance with the observed systematic and body size dependent distribution of the neopulmo in birds.

Considerations of the Problem of the Functional Capacity of the Avian Lung

The avian respiratory apparatus with its differentiation in a rigid gas exchanging portion and a ventilating portion indicates its special functional capacity. Because of the generation of an unidirectional flow of the respiratory air in the paleopulmo which is connected parallel to the primary bronchus, a dead space does not exist in the parabronchial system. It is also lacking in the neopulmo which is directly interposed between primary bronchus and posterior air sacs. Compared to the gas volume of the lung, the volume of the air sacs is very great. The anterior air sacs have a large dead space which continually decreases in the posterior air sacs. Instead, the volume for the ventilation increases which makes up a manyfold of the lung volume despite of the dead space present.

Some measurements of the volume of the air sac space in dead animals have been made using cast preparations (Victorow, 1909; Scharnke, 1938; Zeuthen,

1942; King and Payne, 1958, 1962). Only Dehner (1946) and Scheid and Piiper (1967, 1969) have determined the volume of the air sac space in living ducks and chickens using a wash-out method, additionally the single breath volume (Piiper, Drees, and Scheid, 1970). The number of measurements of the oxygen consumption in different species at rest and in flight is a little greater (Groebbels, 1932, additional literature in Lasiewski, Weathers, and Bernstein, 1967; Tucker, 1968a, b; Piiper, Drees, and Scheid, 1970). Basing on these measurements the inspiratory volume and especially the respiratory minute volume was calculated, or directly measured, respectively. Additionally other species besides poultry were studied, especially budgerigars and hummingbirds. However, our knowledge is still not sufficient.

In the same way unknown as yet are the different anatomical sizes of the avian lung. In the literature it is always reported as a significantly small organ which has the least relative size in the phylum of the vertebrates in relation to body weight (Bethe, 1925; Stresemann, 1927–1934; Portmann, 1950b; Salt and Zeuthen, 1960; Sturkie, 1965). A comparison of the lung weights of birds (summarized by Groebbels, 1932) which vary between 0.8 and 1.7% of the body weight to the known few values of mammals (Gerhartz, 1926; Seeliger, 1960, and orienting measurements of the author) do not show marked differences, however. The "smaller size" of the avian lung is only seemingly smaller than the inflated mammalian lung because of its more compact, denser structure.

Very great differences between the various species can be found in the construction of the individual avian lung. For once the portion of its volume that is occupied by the mantle of respiratory tissue, the network of air and blood capillaries varies in a certain relation to the total mass of parabronchi. In penguins, coots, chickens and mute swans this respiratory tissue occupies only 50% of the parabronchial and thus of the lung volume, while in ducks, pigeons, gulls and buzzards already 65% of the lung volume are filled by respiratory tissue. The greatest values are found in small parakeets and song birds with a 85% share of the respiratory tissue in the lung volume (Duncker, 1969), However, the size of the organ has not been considered in these measurements so that these values cannot be interpreted as relative and absolute values in relation to the total size of the respiratory tissue. This is especially understandable if the chicken is compared to the well flying mute swan. Also the width of the air capillaries which varies between 3 and 10 µ (Oppel, 1905; Stanislaus, 1937) from species to species must be considered. The smaller values are always found in well flying species, the wide air capillaries in species flying poorly or not at all.

Fischer (1905) suggested that the connection of air capillary nets of neighbouring parabronchi has a special functional significance. The connections are present in many well flying species, but also they are lacking in other good flyers like ducks and swans. The connection of the parabronchi via the air capillaries probably has only a slight significance; for in the air capillaries a renewal of the gas composition may not be expected by a flow of gas but only by diffusion. As calculations of Zeuthen (1942) and Hazelhoff (1943, 1951) have shown, a partial pressure gradient of less than 1 mm Hg exists in the mantle of the parabronchi, maximally 500–600 µ thick, from the free lumen as far as into the most distant air capillary. Thereby a sufficient diffusion is guaranteed in the

whole air capillary system. A cross linking of the adjoining parabronchi or a
separation by connective tissue septa seems to have only developmental physiological significance and no functional relevance. On the contrary the total mass
of the respiratory tissue and the size of the air capillaries are of greatest importance
since the size of the exchanging surface is directly related to these factors. These
values very much vary in the different avian species, as can be seen in histological
preparations. Until now only single estimations (Marcus, 1928; Stanislaus, 1937)
exist which gave the following results: 175 cm² exchange surface per gram body
weight for the pigeon, 666 cm² for the hummingbird, compared to values of
11–55 cm² for mammals (from horses to mice). Man has 7 cm², according to
Marcus and 10 cm² exchange area per gram body weight, according to new,
improved calculations based on measurements by Weibel (1963).

First exact measurements corresponding to the method developed by Weibel
(1963) are present for the chicken, the Canada goose and the carrion crow (Duncker,
1971). It was found that the chicken has an effective exchange area of 192 mm²
per mm³ of air-blood capillary network of the parabronchial mantle, the Canada
goose 299 mm²/mm³ and the crow 328 mm²/mm³. For man this value lies, dependent on age, between 18.4 mm² and 25.5 mm² per mm³ alveolar tissue, according to Weibel's (1963) data, thus more than 10 times below the data for avian
lungs. When the values found for the three avian species are related to their
body weights the following results are found: 18.0 cm² exchange area per gram
body weight for the chicken, 22.2 cm²/g for the Canada goose, and for the crow
95.0 cm²/g. In order to interpret these values, numerous measurements on further
species of different size and various flying capacity are needed.

The estimated and the first measured values confirm the impression which
is evoked by the microscopical picture; they prove that the size of the exchange
surface per unit volume of the avian lung is at least 10 times above the mammalian lung in well flying species because of the development of air capillaries.
Between a poor flyer like the chicken and a good flyer like a small migratory
bird a difference of the magnitude of 10 times must also be assumed. Further
quantitative studies of this problem are needed.

An indication of the very different functional capacities of individual species
results from the work of Olander, Burton, and Adler (1967) which demonstrates
a chronic hypoxia and high mortality rate for chickens at 4000 m above sea
level, while sparrows live at 6100 m above sea level with increased metabolism
and are even capable of flying short distances (Tucker, 1968b). Mammals are
moribund at this height where a number of migratory birds fly during their
trip (Lack, 1960; Nisbet, 1963). Besides the great differences from species to
species in the size of the exchange surface a number of other factors play a significant part in the functional capacity of the lung-circulation apparatus, for
instance differences in the capacity of binding oxygen and the affinity of hemoglobin for oxygen, expressed as the tension of half saturation which are specific
to the species. The measurements of Wastl and Leiner (1931), Bartels, Hiller,
and Reinhardt (1966), and Tucker (1968b) show that the oxygen binding capacity
in adult animals varies between 17.0% (ml O_2/100 ml blood) in ducks and carrion
crows via 17.93% in chickens, 19.1% in sparrows, 19.8% in geese and 20.0%
in pigeons. Young chickens have an O_2 capacity of only 9.13–11.5%. The tension

of half-saturation of the blood at P_{CO_2} of 40 mm Hg and at 41–42°C lies at a P_{O_2} of 50 mm Hg, the values for the chicken are greatly deviating. The oxygen dissociation curve is shifted to the right towards higher pressures and has a markedly flatter shape.

The blood flow intensity which perfuses the lung per unit time and which is identical to the cardiac output per minute is another factor that determines the total capacity of the gas exchange. The avian heart is always larger than the heart of mammals of the same size, both in large and in small species, having extreme values in small birds like song birds and hummingbirds of 1.4–2.8% of the body weight (Benninghoff, 1933; Stanislaus, 1937; Portmann, 1950a; Simons, 1960). The heart beat frequency of birds at rest in a number of studies is reported to be higher than that in mammals of comparable size (Lehmann, 1925; Simons, 1960; Lasiewski, Weathers, and Bernstein, 1967; Tucker, 1968b). However, the avian pulse at rest seems to be lower than generally reported and lower than that of comparable mammals according to measurements of birds being definitely at rest (Calder, 1968; Berger, Hart, and Roy, 1970; Berger, personal communication). Consequently, a much larger increase in the maximal minute volume of the heart compared to that at rest would result (Berger, Hart, and Roy, 1970) which could correspond in order of magnitude to the rise of the gas exchange capacity. Consequently the cardiac output per minute is remarkably greater than in comparable mammals.

A characteristic fact for the great functional capacity of the avian lung was first observed by Zeuthen (1942) and later confirmed by Piiper, Pfeifer, and Scheid (1969), Piiper, Drees, and Scheid (1970), Scheid and Piiper (1970): The expiratory air and thus the end parabronchial air has a remarkably higher CO_2-content than the arterialised lung blood. This difference is caused by the construction of the parabronchi as long tubes which are perfused by air in their whole length. The inspiratory air, entering the parabronchi at one end, equilibrates with the blood in the mantle of air and blood capillaries so that the blood has a partial CO_2-pressure just slightly above the CO_2-pressure of the inspiratory air at this level. On its way through the parabronchus the CO_2-content of the air will rise to its final parabronchial value. The blood equilibrates with the partial CO_2-pressure of the respiratory air at the corresponding levels. In relation to the different partial CO_2-pressures in the parabronchus the outflowing blood also has differences in its partial CO_2-pressure, dependent on the level of equilibration. By summation the partial CO_2-pressure of the total arterialised blood lies considerably below that of the expiratory air.

Values like these which seem paradoxical compared to the mammalian lung are shown by the O_2-content of the blood of a chicken only during hypoxis of the inspiratory air (92 mm Hg) (Scheid and Piiper, 1970). Under these conditions the P_{O_2} of the arterial blood is higher than in the end parabronchial air. The question arises whether this is also possible in more efficient birds at normal P_{O_2} of the inspiratory air. However, these values show the enormous advantaee of the construction of a circulating air system with long parabronchi compared to a blindly ending bronchial tree with alveoles in which exchange capacities found in birds are not possible.

The difference between the arterialised blood of the pulmonary vein and the expiratory air must also be related to the extent of lung ventilation and the amount of the O_2-consumption and CO_2-production. The oxygen binding capacity of the hemoglobin and the oxygen dissociation curve determine which amount of oxygen can maximally be exchanged at the given partial pressures. A certain time of contact is necessary for this exchange (ref. to Frech, Schultehinrichs, Vogel, and Thews, 1968). The extent of the exchange at the individual levels and thus the question at which point of the parabronchus the gas exchange maximally possible between blood and air is finished, depends of the flow velocity in the parabronchus. At slow flow velocities end parabronchial value will be reached after only a short stretch, far before the end of the parabronchus, while at high flow velocities the exchange in the initial portion of the parabronchus remains incomplete because of the shortness of the time of contact.

Because of these temporal conditions of the gas exchange very different conditions for the gas exchange at various levels of partial pressure result along the long parabronchus the position of which depends on the flow velocity in the parabronchus. Thereby very different conditions for the gas exchange are given for blood inflowing into the whole parabronchial mantle. In the initial portion an optimal exchange with the inspiratory air is guaranteed; when the end parabronchial value of the gas composition is reached, a further exchange cannot take place anymore, no matter at which level of the parabronchus this value is reached. Corresponding to the extent of the ventilation a variously large part of the blood would have to perfuse the lung without the possibility of a gas exchange. Therefore a variably large shunt should exist in the lung circulation.

It follows from the construction of the bronchial system that the extent of the shunt should be a function of the degree of ventilation. Not until at maximal ventilation an optimal relation between cardiac output per minute and gas exchange should exist because only then all parabronchi are perfused so extensively that a gas exchange may take place along their whole length. During respiration at rest a large shunt should exist in the lung circulation. This should be especially true if the hypothesis, stated in this study, that the paleopulmo is not perfused during respiration at rest when a well developed neopulmo exists, is correct. This is perhaps the reason for the discrepancy between the data of Bartels, Hiller, and Reinhardt (1966) with an oxygen capacity of 17.93% by volume for the adult chicken and those of Morgan and Chichester (1935), Chiodi and Terman (1965) and Piiper, Drees, and Scheid (1970) with an O_2-content of 12.5, 12.7, and 10.0% by volume in the blood of chickens.

Comroe (1968) reports for the mammalian lung that the lowered P_{O_2} in insufficiently ventilated alveolar regions causes a constriction of the arterioles. A number of recent studies concerning this behaviour of the mammalian lung have been made. They prove that the perfusion is drastically lowered at hypoxia and/or hypercapnia in the alveolar air, in the same way as in unventilated parts of the lung (Baer, Howard, McCurrie, and Shaw, 1969; Barer, Howard, and Shaw, 1970; Hauge, 1969; Lloyd, 1966, 1968; Shaw, 1970).

It can well be understood from these data that the unventilated parts of the avian lung are also hardly perfused with blood, a fact which could lead to the reduction of the circulation-shunt necessary for the respiration at rest.

This problem arises in the same manner whether the paleopulmo at rest is perfused a little or not at all. In both cases only the portions of the parabronchi, taking part in the gas exchange are of different size. The construction of long parabronchi necessarily causes the problem of more or less great parts of the parabronchi which do not take part in the gas exchange during respiration at rest. Physiologically, nothing is known about this problem at the moment.

Besides, receptors have been described in the avian lung which react on an increase of the CO_2-content of the respiratory air (Peterson and Fedde, 1968; Ray and Fedde, 1969; Fedde and Peterson, 1970). The receptors are situated in the primary bronchus (Cook and King, 1969 b). Besides, first data of the innervation of the avian lung have been presented (Cook and King, 1969a; McLelland, 1969; Akester and Man, 1969; Burnstock, 1969; Bennett and Malmfors, 1970) as well as numerous data about the nervous control of the respiration in chickens (Fedde and Burger, 1963; Fedde, Burger, and Kitchell, 1963a, b, 1964b; King, Molony, McLelland, Bowsher, and Mortimer, 1968; King, McLelland, Molony, and Mortimer, 1969; King, McLelland, Molony, Bowsher, Mortimer, and White, 1969; Jones, 1969; Richards, 1969; Fedde, 1970). These findings may be summarized: the function of the avian lung is subject to a very differentiated control both by the ventilation and blood perfusion. A part of the factors is the direct reaction of the vessels to changes in the ventilation and the partial pressures in the individual parabronchi, a second, considerable part of factors is the nervous control of the respiration and circulation.

However, a certain shunt of the circulation remains as a special feature of the avian lung during the respiration at rest. This shunt results from the type of construction of the lung of birds. Such a shunt may be compensated only by a rise of the cardiac output per minute. Perhaps this is one physiological reason for the relatively low O_2-content of the arterial blood (Piiper, Drees, and Scheid, 1970) and for the relatively larger hearts and higher pulse frequency of birds at rest, compared to mammals.

During the transition to the maximal functional capacity, the flight, the lung is completely ventilated and the shunt is cancelled. It follows that the changes of the circulation should be considerably smaller during the transition from rest to maximal function than during comparable changes in work in mammals. This may be assumed when the data of the increase of the O_2-consumption during the transition to flight up to the 10-fold (Berger, Hart, and Roy, 1970) the 11- to 20-fold (Tucker, 1968a, 1969), and the 25-fold (Zeuthen, 1942) of the value at rest are compared to the rise of the heart beat frequency up to the 2–3-fold of the normal value. The following conclusions could be drawn: the lung-circulation apparatus of birds which in its functional capacity is characterized by the high values of O_2-consumption, is optimally constructed in relation to its upper functional limit, that maximum stress may be endured as perpetual stress. In order to prove this assumption, the reader is reminded of the migration of many avian species which may last for a few weeks. This construction for a perpetual maximum stress requires an increased circulational effort at rest, however. The specific functional characteristics of the avian lung by which it differs from the lungs of all other vertebrates, are resulting from the special construction of the bronchial system.

Summarily the special functional capacity of the avian lung may be traced back to the following characteristics of construction: The effective exchange surface per unit volume has been increased more than 10 times over that of the mammalian lung by the development of air capillaries instead of alveoles. The resulting construction which is constant in volume, required the development of air sacs as bellows for the lung which permit an extremely effective ventilation of the tube system of the lung. The parabronchi, developed as long tubes, with their exchange principle as multi-capillary-system have physiological exchange capacities which by far exceed those of the mammalian lung and are characterized by a seemingly paradoxical behaviour of a higher P_{CO_2} and, under certain conditions, a lower P_{O_2} in the expiratory air than in the arterialised blood. Together with the special functional capacity of the circulation which finds its expression in a heart size, pulse frequency and cardiac output per minute by far exceeding that of the mammals, and an oxygen dissociation curve of the hemoglobin which is shifted to the right thus allowing a better utilization of the O_2-content of the blood in the tissues, an apparatus has been developed in birds which is fully adapted to long maximum stresses like the migration of birds. The problems which result from this construction, especially the circulation at rest, are totally unknown as yet.

Besides the respiratory function which we know in its outline, the lung air sac system has an important further function which is attributed to it by the lack of sweat glands in this homoiothermous vertebrate group. Water is steadily evaporated by the change of respiratory air. At increased respiration during long flights this loss of water may already become a limiting element (Nisbet, 1963; Nisbet, Drury, and Baird, 1963). Additionally, this makes possible the increase of water evaporation and thereby a heat regulatory function by raising the respiration above the amount necessary for the gas exchange. This was studied by Soum (1896), Victorow (1909), Kayser (1930), von Saalfeld (1936), Scharnke (1938), Kendeigh (1944), and Salt (1964) and in recent years by MacMillen and Trost (1967), Lasiewski, Weathers, and Bernstein (1967), Breitenbach and Baskett (1967), Crawford and Schmidt-Nielsen (1967), Calder and Schmidt-Nielsen (1967, 1968), Hart and Roy (1967), Tucker (1968a), Schmidt-Nielsen, Hainsworth, and Murrish (1970). However, other structures of the bird, like the inferior surface of the wing which is unfolded in flight and has only few feathers, and the unfeathered legs with their very well controllable capillary net (Steen and Steen, 1965) are of great importance for the temperature regulation.

Functional Characterization of the Avian Lung Compared to the Mammalian Lung

As the considerations of the functional capacity of the avian lung have shown, a number of factors which are based on the structure of the avian lung, determine the capacity of exchange which make possible such a long migration. The development of a rigid, volume constant lung permits the development of an air and blood capillary net in a considerable thickness around the individual parabronchial lumen. Air capillaries would collapse during variations of the volume, and an unfolding during an expansion of the lung would become impossible because of the great surface tension. An enormous enlargement of the exchange surface was achieved by the development of the air capillaries. The exchange area per unit volume is more than 10 times larger in well flying species than in a mammalian lung. The air capillaries are only 3–10 μ wide, occupying about 50–80% of the parabronchial volume, while the diameter of mammalian alveoles varies between 35 and 500 μ (Tenney and Remmers, 1963; Spells, 1968).

On the other hand, a rigid lung also allows the development of a tube system perfused by flow dynamic regulation. Together with the inseparable air sac system a relatively much larger respiratory volume may be drawn through the lung in the individual respiratory phases, thus corresponding to the size of the exchange surface. In the mammalian lung gas exchanging and ventilating apparatus are not separated, causing on one hand the limitation of the exchange surface because of the alveolar size which has a minimal diameter of 35 μ, and on the other hand mostly a larger functional dead space and a considerable residual volume.

Additionally, in mammals the alveolar size is very much dependent on the size of the animal, ranging from 35 μ to well over 500 μ, while the avian air capillaries vary only between 3 and 10 μ. Not only an absolute lower size limit but also a lower size limit relative to the body size is existent in mammals. In a very large lung with very small alveoles the afferent bronchi would necessarily be much more numerous and narrower. Thereby the flow resistance for the ventilation of the lung would rise so considerably that the exchange surface of the mammalian lung is significantly limited in large animals (because of these relations). A diminution of the alveoles and therefore an enlargement of the exchange surface is only possible in small mammals. In birds, however, the parabronchial lumen in its width must be adapted to the animal size because of the flow resistance increasing with the length, but not the width of their capillaries. For in the air capillaries the gas exchange takes place only by diffusion. Thus the exchange surface may be increased even in large birds almost independent of the body size.

The perfusion of the parabronchi in one direction — in the paleopulmo always unidirectional, in the neopulmo changing with the inspiratory phases — renders possible that the partial CO_2-pressure in the arterialised blood lies below and the partial O_2-pressure above that of the expiratory air, inspite of the admixture of shunt blood. This is impossible in the mammalian lung. Together with the O_2-dissociation curve of the hemoglobin, shifted to the right, and thereby the better utilization of the O_2-content of the blood in the tissues, very effective means of supply have been developed in birds.

Large exchange surfaces and high efficiency of the O_2-exchange in the lung and in the tissues are the decisive requirements for the long time maximum stresses of birds, the second side of which is determined by the circulation. For such maximum stresses the 25-fold of the metabolism at rest has been reported as the maximal value (Zeuthen, 1942) while for a number of other species the 10-fold (Berger, Hart, and Roy, 1970) up to the 11- to 20-fold (Tucker, 1968a, 1969) of the metabolism at rest have been found as maximal values. As long time functional capacities these values by far exceed those possible in mammals.

With the development of the neopulmo a differentiation of the gas exchanging portion of the respiratory apparatus in two structurally and functionally different parts has taken place in systematically higher species. The neopulmo alone is probably responsible for the respiration at rest, while neopulmo and paleopulmo cooperate in the respiration during stress. Such a differentiation is not possible in the mammalian lung because of its construction. They possess a general, not differentiable lung structure which lacks the development in a ventilating and a gas exchanging apparatus and therefore the development of structures for perpetual maximum stresses.

The differentiation of the locomotor systems of the avian body has made the wing muscles independent of those of the thorax and of the abdomen so that flight and respiratory motions may be performed independent of each other. This has a special importance for the avian evolution because wing beat frequency and respiratory frequency are both related to body size, however, in a very different manner. Only in birds of the size of pigeons, both frequencies are identical in flight; smaller birds have a lesser respiratory than wing beat frequency, larger a higher respiratory frequency. Because of the independence of the loco- motor systems it became possible to develop the variety of the different avian body sizes. Contrary to mammals, birds are lacking auxiliary respiratory muscles. Instead, their inspiratory muscles are extensively developed, the degree of effi- ciency of the Mm. intercostales externi with their insertions at the uncinate processes so characteristic for birds, is increased. Not only the avian lung but in the same way also the locomotor system shows a high degree of differentiation. Both of them together allow the high functional capacity in the various avian species.

The avian respiratory apparatus is characterized by the fact that the actual lung, consistent of the parabronchi does not possess a dead space. The residual volume, however, is large; it includes the air content of the total bronchial system. The air sacs have a large dead space which considerably decreases from the anterior to the posterior air sacs. In the posterior air sacs which serve the ventilation, a certain part of them is still dead space so that dead space air is admixed to the expiratory air. Because of the large dead space, especially in the anterior air sacs, and the residual volume of the whole bronchial system, birds cannot dive deep or for a long time; not considering the problem of the buoyancy, they are subject to compression of the trunk and Caisson's disease at greater depths. They are restricted to the air sphere.

Generally, the mammals differ in their variability of their lung volume; whales as a specific example are able to decrease the residual volume of their lungs by a horizontal displacement of their diaphragm to such an extent that all alveoles collapse completely; individual species may dive more than 1 000 m deep and for almost 2 hours (Andersen, 1966). Thereby they avoid not only the danger of a thorax compression under the high pressure and Caisson's disease, but they may also surface very quickly and inspire by the strong unfolding of the lung 90% or more of the total volume fresh air and compensate the oxygen debt acquired during the long dive in a very short time.

Birds, because of their enormously increased exchange surface and the high efficiency of the gas exchange due to the multi-capillary-flow system (Scheid and Piiper, 1968, 1970) are not only able to live in heights above 5000 m, but some species even rise to this height for their migration, a long time maximum stress. All anatomical and physiological data about these species are lacking as yet so that we are able to understand these performances only from the qualitative basic principle of construction of the avian lung, not however, how especially individual species obtain these characteristics. Thus the most important question remains unanswered: what physiological consequences and also facilitations has a flight in such a height?

The special structure of the respiratory apparatus of birds — contrary to the mammals — is also expressed by the dependence from the special conditions of the avian ontogenesis. Because of the basic construction of the immobil incorporation into an incompressible thoracic cavity which is based on the constructive necessities of the air capillary structure, the avian lung does not have the possibility to unfold at birth, as it is typical for the mammal. The avian lung must be developed as a rigid, air filled tube system before it takes up its respiratory function.

Therefore the development of the birds within the egg is a necessary requirement for the development of the complicatedly structured respiratory apparatus. At the end of the development, according to the duration of the egg development 2–5 days before hatching the embryos have ingested the amniotic fluid and the rest of the egg white united with it (Romanoff, 1960). Not until then a very marked development of the quantitatively relatively underdeveloped lung sets in and together with it regular respiratory motions. Shortly afterwards, $1^1/_2$ to 4 days before hatching the membrane separating the air bubble of the egg is pierced through and from now on the embryo lies in the air filled amniotic cavity (Romanoff, 1960; Vince and Salter, 1967; Visschedijk, 1968a, b, c).

With the first respiratory motions the large posterior air sacs, important for the ventilation which are already developed, are unfolded. With the respiratory motions which now become regular and deeper, the tubular parabronchial system is ventilated. Then the development of the first layer of air capillaries around the parabronchial volume begins (Petrik, 1967) interlacing with the developing blood capillaries. Thus the air capillaries which cannot be unfolded are developed already at their beginning starting from an air filled parabronchial lumen. During this time the oxygen supply of the embryo is still guaranteed by the functioning chorioallantois. The respiratory apparatus is differentiated under functioning air respiration in its last phase of development, without having to guarantee the oxygen supply of the embryo. For the lung attains the ability for gas exchange only by the development of the air capillaries with the help of air respiration. At the time of hatching it may then overtake the gas exchange and substitute the chorioallantois. From these absolutely necessary conditions it is understandable that no bird was able to develop viviparously, an unique case in the whole tribe of vertebrates.

The respiratory apparatus of birds and mammals is remarkably characterized by the conditions of its ontogenetical development, especially since it has a central importance for these two classes which are homoiothermous and fundamentally differ from all other classes by an intensive and high metabolism which serves the regulation of temperature.

In the foregoing it could be shown that a number of functional consequences accompany the ontogenetically strongly influenced differentiation in these two different types of the respiratory apparatus. The birds, with their specifically developed ventilation through their tube lung and with the development of air capillaries could not only attain an enormous enlargement of the exchange surface but also a high degree of efficiency of the gas exchange which permits the maximum stress of the flight for a long time and also in great heights. They are not able to dive for a longer time or into greater depths, however. Mammals with horizontal diaphragms on the contrary have the possibility to almost totally eliminate the residual volume so that they were able to adapt to diving for a long time and into greater depths. With a great enlargement of the respiratory apparatus the development of flight was also made possible in the group of the insectivora. Their flight capacity, however, was limited to low heights, lesser performance and to species which do not reach the size of large birds.

Summary

The purpose of this study is the elaboration of a concept of the lung air sac system basing on comparative and functional anatomical investigations which may serve as the basis of further physiological studies. Using a specially devised injection technique more than 500 birds of 150 species, from penguins to song birds, were injected with silicon-rubber. In this manner the lung air sac system was demonstrated in connection with the skeleton and then prepared considering the lung construction and the connection of the air sacs. Additionally, 45 species after fixation were prepared in the usual manner. The microscopical structure of the lung air sac system was studied on membrane preparations of the air sac walls and on histological sections through the lung.

1) Studying the locomotor system of the birds it was found that the action of the locomotor system of the trunk is independent from those of the wings and of the legs. Thus a complete dissociation of flight and respiratory motions is realized. Because of the lack of auxiliary respiratory muscles, the inspiratory muscles have to be developed especially strong. This is especially accomplished by the more efficient lever arm for those parts of the Mm. intercostales externi which insert at the well developed uncinate processes of the ribs. All muscles of the abdomen, besides the corresponding thoracic muscles have an expiratory function. It is characteristic for birds that the expiration is performed by muscle actions in all phases.

2) The lungs are grown together with the dorsal thoracic cavity at all sides, they do not possess a pleural cleft. Besides, they are displaced towards dorsal as far as directly beneath the transverse processes of the vertebrae so that they enclose the ribs which pass arc-like to the vertebral column, in deep incisures. Because of the strutting of the ribs the avian thorax is not transversely compressible. The anterior ribs perform a pure forward motion, likewise the upper parts of the caudal ribs. The space for the lungs, ventrally limited by the horizontal septum, is subject to only small changes in volume during respiration which are compensated by the action of the Mm. costopulmonales. The avian lung therefore is a rigid structure practically constant in volume.

3) The sternum performs a hinge-like motion during respiration by which the air sacs, contrary to the lung, are changed in their volume, increasingly towards caudal. By the connection of the posterior thoracic and the abdominal air sac to a large laterobronchus and the primary bronchus, respectively, these air sacs obtain the function of bellows for the ventilation of the lung. The anterior air sacs (cervical, impar interclavicular and anterior thoracic air sac) are of only small importance for the respiration.

4) The constancy in volume of the lung is the necessary requirement for the development of air capillaries. With their small diameter (3–10 μ) they have such a sharp curvature that their surface tension at the moistened tissue surface to air is considerably greater than in the mammalian lung alveoles the smallest of which measure 35 μ in diameter. The surface film of phospholipids which is also developed in the air capillaries, is not capable of reducing the surface tension to such an extent as in mammalian alveoles so that an unfolding by muscular forces would be possible. Therefore, air capillaries are existent only as rigid tubes, this is guaranteed by a lung constant in volume. The surface film of the air capillaries has the purpose of reducing the surface tension to such an extent that a transudation may not take place and thus close the air capillaries. The exchange surface per unit volume is enlarged to more than 10 times that of the mammalian lung by the air capillaries; to a certain extent, differences are found between the various avian species. — The air capillaries form a closely interlaced network with the blood capillaries, one net just filling the interstices of the other. This blood-air capillary network forms the mantle of the parabronchi, 300–600 μ thick, in which a gas exchange takes place from the parabronchial lumen only by diffusion. The parabronchi are the long stretched, smallest bronchial units of the avian lung, being connected on both ends to secondary bronchi. A blindly ending bronchial tree is not existent in the avian lung.

5) The rest of the bronchial system is also developed as a mainly rigid tube system in the lung of constant volume. The primary bronchus gives off the first group of secondary bronchi, the four ventrobronchi, directly after its entrance into the lung. The ventrobronchi spread across the whole ventral surface of the lung and ramify. The primary bronchus then passes as the vestibulum free of branches to the lateral surface of the lung and bends towards caudal. Just above the inferior lung margin it runs to the caudal lung tip and terminates into the abdominal air sac. During its course at the lung surface it gives off the second group of secondary bronchi, the seven to ten dorsobronchi, which spread at the dorsolateral lung surface. The dorsobronchi are connected to the ventrobronchi through a dense, long stretched network of parabronchi. In the parabronchi, more exactly in their mantle of air and blood capillaries the gas exchange takes place. In the compact network of parabronchi which is enclosed between the superficial layers of the ventrobronchi and dorsobronchi like the filling of a sandwich, the vascular tree of the lung is spread out, independent of the course of the primary and secondary bronchus. This bronchial system is therefore connected parallel to the primary bronchus. It is well developed in all birds, and in penguins, emus, cormorants and storks it occupies the whole or almost the whole lung. This bronchial system with its respiratory tissue is described as the "paleopulmo".

6) Opposite to the dorsobronchi, towards ventral, a small group of secondary bronchi arises, the laterobronchi. The first or second leads into the posterior thoracic air sac as a short, sturdy stem, the rest of the laterobronchi connect through their parabronchi to the ventrobronchi. While the posterior air sacs in penguins, emus, cormorants and storks are almost completely connected through the wide laterobronchus and primary bronchus, a parabronchial net originates from the primary and laterobronchus which opens into the posterior air sacs, too, as it is found in birds with a higher systematical position. If this network is better developed, it includes also the initial portions of the dorsobronchi and then opens not anymore into the ostia of the primary and laterobronchus into the air sacs but into saccobronchi of its own. This parabronchial net which is directly interposed between primary bronchus and posterior air sacs, is termed the "neopulmo". The development of the neopulmo reaches such an extent that it almost totally takes over the connection of the posterior air sacs in pigeons, fowllike and song birds. The primary bronchus becomes so narrow that it is abolished functionally in its caudal portion; a wide laterobronchus, however, always remains. The neopulmo occupies the laterocaudal part of the lung and constitutes never more than 20% of the total parabronchial mass of the lung.

7) The very constant construction of the paleopulmo in the whole class of birds suggests that this parallel bronchial system is perfused in the same direction during inspiration and expiration, according to Hazelhoff's theory. This theory agrees with the angles of ramification and the relations of the cross sectional areas observed in this study and indicates that an unidirectional air flow out of the primary bronchus into the dorsobronchi and through the parabronchi into the ventrobronchi leads back into the primary bronchus during inspiration *and* expiration. Such a flow dynamic regulation has a limiting value of the flow velocity in the primary bronchus, because of the flow resistance in the parallel system which must be overcome. Below this limiting value this kind of ventilation is not possible anymore.

8) These requirements do not exist for the neopulmo which directly connects primary bronchus and posterior air sacs. It will be ventilated in changing directions during inspiration and expiration even under very small differences in pressure. Thus the hypothesis is stated that the neopulmo in systematically higher species could solely maintain the respiration at rest. With the transition to deeper respiration automatically the paleopulmo is also ventilated which then, as the larger part of the lung functions in the gas exchange together with the neopulmo during maximum stresses as for instance in flight.

9) Independent of this hypothesis a study of the gas exchange in the long stretched parabronchi shows that great local differences in the arterialisation of the blood exist in the avian lung. This would indicate a circulation shunt related to the ventilation value in the lung which, according to present knowledge of the mammalian lung could be lowered drastically by autoregulation. The assumption of a certain shunt of the circulation is supported by the fact that birds have considerably greater relative heart weights and an equally higher heart beat frequency at rest than comparable mammals. Therefore, a markedly greater cardiac output per minute at rest must result, which could serve to compensate the circulation shunt. Not until maximal respiration this circulation

shunt is completely abolished; for this a lesser increase of the circulatory capacity is necessary as it would correspond to the increase of the gas exchange. Thus the avian lung with its circulatory apparatus seems to be constructed for the purpose of accomplishing perpetual maximum stress under optimal conditions.

10) The development of air capillaries and the resulting enormous enlargement of the exchange surface is dependent on the rigidity of the tubes of the bronchial system and on the other hand on the flow dynamic regulation of the ventilation. This system which is incorporated into the incompressible thorax cannot be unfolded at the moment of birth. Thus the development of the avian lung is connected to the development of the embryo within the egg. It allows the ventilation of the lungs and air sacs with the help of the air bubble in the last 2–5 days before hatching and the development of the first layer of air capillaries in the parabronchial wall at simultaneous air respiration, while gas exchange still is maintained by the chorioallantois. With the lung ready for function which may overtake the gas exchange, the chicken hatches. The functional significance of these procedures may be concluded from the fact that the highly developed class of birds has not developed a single viviparous species, contrary to all other classes of vertebrates. — In comparison, the mammalian lung is constructed in such a manner to be unfolded at birth. However, thereby a higher limiting value of the diameter for unfoldable alveoles which cannot be undercut, is fixed, limiting the total size of the gas exchange surface for mammals. They are never able to develop the more than ten times larger exchange surface of the birds which is the requirement for performances as the flight at great heights or the continual migration for days or weeks.

Das Lungen-Luftsacksystem der Vögel

Zusammenfassung

Das Ziel dieser Arbeit ist, ein Konzept der Funktion des Lungen-Luftsacksystems auf Grund vergleichend- und funktionell-anatomischer Untersuchungen zu erarbeiten, das als Basis weiterer, auch physiologischer Untersuchungen dienen kann. Mit Hilfe einer besonderen Injektionstechnik wurden über 500 Vögel aus 150 Arten, von den Pinguinen bis zu den Singvögeln, mit Silicon-Kautschuk injiziert. Damit wurde das Lungen-Luftsacksystem im Zusammenhang mit dem Skelet dargestellt und im Anschluß daran im Hinblick auf den Aufbau der Lunge und den Anschluß der Luftsäcke präparatorisch zerlegt. Daneben wurden 45 Arten in üblicher Weise nach einer Fixierung präpariert. An Häutchenpräparaten der Luftsackwandungen und an Schnitten durch die Lungen wurde der mikroskopische Bau des Bronchialsystems untersucht.

1. Beim Studium des Bewegungsapparates der Vögel zeigt sich, daß die Tätigkeit des Bewegungssystems des Rumpfes ganz unabhängig ist von denen des Flügels und des Beines. Dadurch ist die völlige Dissoziation von Flug- und Atembewegungen möglich. Durch das Fehlen einer Atemhilfsmuskulatur muß die Inspirationsmuskulatur besonders kräftig ausgebildet sein. Das ist vor allem durch den wirksameren Hebelarm für die an den gut entwickelten Processus uncinati der Rippen ansetzenden Teile der Mm. intercostales externi gegeben.

Exspiratorisch wirken neben den betreffenden Thoraxmuskeln alle Muskeln des Abdomen. Charakteristisch für die Vögel ist eine in allen Phasen durch Muskeltätigkeit aktive Exspiration.

2. Die Lungen sind im dorsalen Thoraxraum allseitig verwachsen, sie besitzen keinen Pleuraspalt. Außerdem sind sie nach dorsal bis direkt unter die Processus transversi der Wirbel verlagert, so daß sie die bogenförmig an die Wirbelsäule ziehenden Rippen in tiefen Einschnitten einschließen. Durch die Verstrebung der Rippen ist der Vogelthorax nicht querkompressibel. Die vorderen Rippen führen reine Vorwärtsbewegungen aus, ebenso die oberen Teile der hinteren Rippen. Der durch das horizontale Septum ventral abgegrenzte Raum für die Lungen führt während der Atmung nur geringfügige Volumenänderungen aus, die durch die Tätigkeit der Mm. costopulmonales kompensiert werden. Die Vogellunge ist dadurch ein praktisch volumenkonstantes, starres Gebilde.

3. Das Sternum führt bei der Atmung eine Scharnierbewegung aus, durch die im Gegensatz zur Lunge die Luftsäcke nach caudal zunehmend in ihrem Volumen verändert werden. Durch den Anschluß des hinteren thorakalen und des abdominalen Luftsackes an einen großen Laterobronchus bzw. an den Hauptbronchus erhalten diese Säcke die Funktion von Blasebälgen für die Ventilation der Lunge. Die vorderen Luftsäcke (cervicaler, unpaarer interclavicularer und vorderer thorakaler Luftsack) besitzen dagegen für die Atmung eine nur geringe Bedeutung.

4. Die Volumenkonstanz der Lunge ist die notwendige Voraussetzung für die Ausbildung von Luftcapillaren. Sie besitzen mit ihrem geringen Durchmesser (3—10 μ) eine so scharfe Krümmung, daß in ihnen die Oberflächenspannung an der befeuchteten Grenzfläche Gewebe-Luft sehr viel größer ist als in den Alveolen der Säugerlunge, deren kleinste 35 μ im Querschnitt messen. Der auch in den Luftcapillaren gut ausgebildete Oberflächenfilm aus Phospholipiden ist nicht in der Lage, die Oberflächenspannung wie in den Säugeralveolen soweit herabzusetzen, daß eine Entfaltung mit Muskelkräften möglich wäre. Deshalb sind Luftcapillaren nur als starre Röhren existent, was durch eine volumenkonstante Lunge gewährleistet wird. Der Oberflächenfilm der Luftcapillaren besitzt die Aufgabe, die Oberflächenspannung soweit herabzusetzen, daß keine Transsudation auftritt und die Luftcapillaren dadurch nicht zuquellen. Durch die Luftcapillaren wird die Austauschoberfläche pro Volumeneinheit um mehr als eine Zehnerpotenz vergrößert im Vergleich zur Säugerlunge; dabei gibt es in einem gewissen Ausmaß Unterschiede zwischen den verschiedenen Vogelarten. — Die Luftcapillaren bilden zusammen mit Blutcapillaren ein innig vermaschtes Netzwerk, in dem ein Netz stets gerade die Lücken des anderen ausfüllt. Dieses Blut-Luftcapillarnetzwerk bildet den 300—600 μ dicken Mantel der Parabronchien, in dem vom Parabronchiallumen aus nur durch Diffusion ein Gaswechsel erfolgt. Die Parabronchien sind die langgestreckten kleinsten Bronchialeinheiten der Vogellunge, die an beiden Enden mit Sekundärbronchien verbunden sind. Es gibt also in der Vogellunge keinen blind endenden Bronchialbaum.

5. In der volumenkonstanten Lunge ist auch das übrige Bronchialsystem als ein weitgehend starres Röhrenwerk ausgebildet. Der Hauptbronchus gibt direkt nach seinem Eintritt in die Lunge die erste Gruppe der sekundären Bronchien,

die vier Ventrobronchien ab, die sich auf der ganzen ventralen Oberfläche der Lunge ausbreiten und verzweigen. Der Hauptbronchus läuft dann als Vestibulum frei von abgehenden Ästen zu der lateralen Oberfläche der Lunge und biegt dort nach caudal um. Über der Lungenunterkante zieht er zum Lungenende und mündet in den abdominalen Luftsack. Während des Verlaufes an der Oberfläche der Lunge gibt er die zweite Gruppe sekundärer Bronchien, die 7—10 Dorsobronchien ab, die sich auf der latero-dorsalen Oberfläche der Lunge ausbreiten. Die Dorsobronchien sind durch ein dichtes langgestrecktes Netzwerk von Parabronchien mit den Ventrobronchien verbunden. In den Parabronchien mit ihrem Mantel aus Luft- und Blutcapillaren findet der Gasaustausch statt. — In dem kompakten Netzwerk der Parabronchien, das wie die Füllung eines „Sandwich" von den oberflächlichen Lagen der Ventro- bzw. Dorsobronchien zusammengefaßt wird, breitet sich der Gefäßbaum der Lunge aus, unabhängig vom Verlauf des Haupt- und der Sekundärbronchien. Das Bronchialsystem ist also im Nebenschluß an den Hauptbronchus angeschlossen. Es ist bei allen Vögeln gut entwickelt und macht bei Pinguinen, Emus, Kormoranen und Störchen die ganze oder fast die ganze Lunge aus. Dieses Bronchialsystem mit seinem respiratorischen Gewebe wird als „Palaeopulmo" beschrieben.

6. Den Dorsobronchien gegenüber, also nach ventral, entspringt eine kleine Gruppe sekundärer Bronchien, die Laterobronchien. Der erste oder zweite führt als kurzer, kräftiger Stamm in den hinteren thorakalen Luftsack; die übrigen Laterobronchien senden ihre Parabronchien den Ventrobronchien entgegen. Während bei Pinguinen, Emus, Kormoranen und Störchen die hinteren Luftsäcke fast ausschließlich über den weitlumigen Latero- und Hauptbronchus angeschlossen werden, entspringt bei Vögeln mit zunehmend höherer systematischer Stellung von Haupt- und Laterobronchien ein Parabronchialnetz, das ebenfalls in die hinteren Luftsäcke mündet. Bei stärkerer Entwicklung erfaßt dieses Netzwerk auch die Anfangsstrecken der Dorsobronchien und mündet dann auch nicht mehr in den Ostien des Haupt- und Laterobronchus in die Luftsäcke, sondern mit eigenen Saccobronchien. Dieses Parabronchialnetz, das im Hauptschluß zwischen Hauptbronchus und hintere Luftsäcke eingeschaltet ist, wird „Neopulmo" genannt. Die Entwicklung der Neopulmo geht so weit, daß sie bei Tauben, Hühner- und Singvögeln den Anschluß der hinteren Luftsäcke weitgehend übernimmt. Der Hauptbronchus wird so eng, daß er caudal funktionell fortfällt; ein weiter Laterobronchus bleibt dagegen immer bestehen. Die Neopulmo nimmt den laterocaudalen Teil der Lunge ein und umfaßt nie mehr als 20% der gesamten Parabronchienmasse der Lunge.

7. Auf Grund des sehr konstanten Baues der Palaeopulmo in der ganzen Vogelreihe konnte wahrscheinlich gemacht werden, daß dieses Nebenschlußsystem bei In- und Exspiration in gleicher Richtung nach der Theorie von Hazelhoff durchströmt wird. Diese Theorie stimmt mit den in dieser Untersuchung beobachteten Abgangswinkeln und Querschnittsverhältnissen überein und führt zu der Auffassung, daß eine gleichgerichtete Strömung aus dem Hauptbronchus in die Dorsobronchien und über die Parabronchien und Ventrobronchien in den Hauptbronchus bei In- *und* Exspiration zurückführt. Eine solche strömungsdynamische Steuerung hat aber wegen des zu überwindenden Strömungswiderstandes im Nebenschlußsystem einen Grenzwert der Strömungsgeschwindigkeit

im Hauptbronchus, unterhalb dessen diese Art der Belüftung nicht mehr statt-
finden kann.

8. Diese Bedingungen bestehen aber nicht für die Neopulmo, die im Hauptschluß Hauptbronchus und hintere Luftsäcke verbindet. Sie wird bei In- und
Exspiration in wechselnden Richtungen auch bei sehr geringen Druckdifferenzen
durchströmt werden. Daraus wird die Hypothese abgeleitet, daß die Neopulmo
bei den systematisch höher stehenden Formen allein die Ruheatmung unterhalten
könnte. Mit dem Übergang zu stärkeren Atemexkursionen wird dann automatisch
auch die Palaeopulmo ventiliert, die als größerer Lungenteil dann zusammen mit
der Neopulmo den Gasaustausch bei der Höchstleistung wie dem Flug durchführt.

9. Unabhängig von dieser Hypothese ergibt sich aus der Betrachtung der
Gasaustauschvorgänge in den langgestreckten Parabronchien, daß in der Vogellunge, solange keine maximale Atmung erfolgt, große lokale Unterschiede für
die Arterialisierung des Blutes bestehen. Das würde einen von der Ventilations-
größe abhängenden Kreislaufkurzschluß in der Lunge bedeuten, der, nach den
bisherigen Kenntnissen von der Säugerlunge, aber autoregulatorisch drastisch
gesenkt werden könnte. Die Vermutung eines gewissen Kreislaufshunts wird ge-
stützt durch die Tatsache, daß Vögel gegenüber vergleichbaren Säugetieren stets
viel höhere relative Herzgewichte und eine ebenfalls höhere Herzruhefrequenz
besitzen. Zusammen müßte sich daraus ein wesentlich größeres Herzminuten-
volumen in der Ruhe ergeben, das dazu dienen könnte, den Kreislaufkurzschluß
zu kompensieren. Erst bei maximaler Atmung wird der Kreislaufkurzschluß ganz
aufgehoben; dazu ist dann aber eine geringere Steigerung der Kreislaufleistung
notwendig, als es der Steigerung des Gasaustausches entsprechen würde. Danach
scheint die Vogellunge mit ihrem Kreislaufapparat darauf hin konstruiert zu sein,
Dauerhöchstleistungen unter optimalen Bedingungen zu erbringen.

10. Die Ausbildung von Luftcapillaren und die damit gegebene enorme Ober-
flächenvergrößerung sind ebenso wie die strömungsdynamische Steuerung der
Ventilation der Palaeopulmo davon abhängig, daß das Bronchialsystem ein starres
Röhrenwerk ist. Dieses in den nicht kompressiblen Thorax eingefügte System
kann nun aber auch im Geburtsmoment nicht entfaltet werden. Deshalb ist die
Ausbildung der Vogellunge gebunden an eine Entwicklung im Ei. Sie gestattet es,
daß die Lungen und Luftsäcke in den letzten 2—5 Tagen vor dem Schlüpfen
mit Hilfe der Gasblase schon belüftet werden und daß unter bereits ablaufender
Luftatmung die erste Lage von Luftcapillaren in der Wand der Parabronchien
ausgebildet wird, während der Gasaustausch noch von der Chorioallantois durch-
geführt wird. Mit funktionsfähig ausgebildeter Lunge, die den Gasaustausch
übernehmen kann, schlüpft dann das Küken. Die funktionelle Bedeutung dieser
Vorgänge läßt sich daran ablesen, daß die hochentwickelte Gruppe der Vögel
keine einzige lebendgebärende Form ausgebildet hat, im Gegensatz zu allen
anderen Wirbeltiergruppen. — Im Vergleich dazu ist die Säugerlunge daraufhin
konstruiert, bei der Geburt entfaltet werden zu können. Damit ist aber eine
untere, nicht zu unterschreitende Größengrenze für entfaltbare Alveolen gegeben,
die für die Säuger die Gesamtgröße der Austauschoberfläche limitiert. Sie können
nie die um eine Zehnerpotenz größeren Austauschoberflächen der Vögel ausbilden,
die erst die Voraussetzung für Leistungen wie den Flug in großen Höhen oder
den Wanderflug über Tage und Wochen darstellen.

References

Akester, A. R.: The comparative anatomy of the respiratory pathways in the domestic fowl (*Gallus domesticus*), pigeon (*Columba livia*), and domestic duck (*Anas platyrhyncha*). J. Anat. (Lond.) 94, 487–505 (1960).

— Osmiophilic inclusion bodies as the source of laminated membrane in the epithelial lining of avian tertiary bronchi. J. Anat. (Lond.) 107, 189–190 (1970).

— Mann, S. P.: Ultrastructure and innervation of the tertiary-bronchial unit in the lung of *Gallus domesticus*. J. Anat. (Lond.) 105, 202–204 (1969).

Alexander, W. B., Niethammer, G.: Die Vögel der Meere. Hamburg-Berlin: Parey 1959.

Andersen, H. T.: Physiological adaptations in diving vertebrates. Physiol. Rev. 46, 212–243 (1966).

Babak, E.: Die Mechanik und Innervation der Atmung. XVII. Vögel. In: Winterstein, Handbuch der vergleichenden Physiologie, Bd. 1/2, S. 880–950. Jena: Fischer 1921.

Baer, M.: Beiträge zur Kenntnis der Anatomie und Physiologie der Atemwerkzeuge bei den Vögeln. Tübinger Zool. Arb. 2, 87–166 (1896).

— Beiträge zur Kenntnis der Anatomie und Physiologie der Atemwerkzeuge bei den Vögeln. Z. wiss. Zool. 61, 420–498 (1896).

Barer, G. R., Howard, P., McCurrie, J. R., Shaw, J. W.: The mechanism reducing blood flow through unventilated lung. J. Physiol. (Lond.) 200, 67 P (1969).

— — Shaw, J. W.: Sensitivity of pulmonary vessels to hypoxia and hypercapnia. J. Physiol. (Lond.) 206, 25 P (1970).

Bargmann, W., Knoop, A.: Elektronenmikroskopische Untersuchungen an der Reptilien- und Vogellunge. Z. Zellforsch. 54, 541–548 (1961).

Bartels, H., Hiller, G., Reinhardt, W.: Oxygen affinity of chicken blood before and after hatching. Resp. Physiol. 1, 345–356 (1966).

Beddard, F. E.: Notes on the visceral anatomy of birds. No 1. On the so-called omentum. Proc. Zool. Soc. Lond. 1885, 836–844.

— Note on the air-sacs of the Cassowary. Proc. Zool. Soc. Lond. 1886 (a), 145–146.

— On some points in the anatomy of *Chauna chavaria*. Proc. Zool. Soc. Lond. 1886 (b), 178–181.

— Notes on the visceral anatomy of birds. II. On the respiratory organs in certain diving birds. Proc. Zool. Soc. Lond. 1888, 252–258.

— On the oblique septa ("Diaphragm" of Owen) in the passerines and in some other birds. Proc. Zool. Soc. Lond. 1896, 225–231.

— The structure and classification of birds. London: Longmans, Green & Co. 1898.

Beerens, J.: Contribution à l'étude de la respiration des oiseaux. Ann. Physiol. Physicochim. biol. 8, 839–869 (1932).

Bellairs, A. d' A., Jenkin, C. R.: The skeleton of birds. In: Marshall, Biology and comparative physiology of birds, vol. 1, p. 241–300. New York-London: Academic Press 1960.

Bennett, T., Malmfors, T.: The adrenergic nervous system of the domestic fowl (*Gallus domesticus* (L.)). Z. Zellforsch. 106, 22–50 (1970).

Benninghoff, A.: Das Herz. In: Bolk, Göppert, Kallius, Lubosch, Handbuch der vergleichenden Anatomie der Wirbeltiere, Bd. 6, S. 467–556. Berlin-Wien: Urban & Schwarzenberg 1933.

Berger, A. J.: The musculature. In: Marshall, Biology and comparative physiology of birds, vol. 1, p. 301–344. New York-London: Academic Press 1960.

Berger, M., Hart, J. S., Roy, O. Z.: Respiration, oxygen consumption and heart rate in some birds during rest and flight. Z. vergl. Physiol. 66, 200–214 (1970).

— Roy, O. Z., Hart, J. S.: The co-ordination between respiration and wing beats in birds. Z. vergl. Physiol. 66, 190–200 (1970).

Berndt, R., Meise, W.: Naturgeschichte der Vögel, Bd. 1, Allgemeine Vogelkunde. Stuttgart: Franckh'sche Verlagsbuchhandlung 1959.

Bertelli, D.: Contributo alla morfologia ed alla sviluppo del diaframma ornitico. Monit. zool. ital. 9 (1898), cit. to Poole 1909.

— Richerche di embriologia e di anatomia comparata sul diaframma e sull' apparechio respiratorio dei vertebrati. Arch. ital. Anat. Embriol. 4, 593–633 and 776–844 (1905).

Bethe, A.: Atmung: Allgemeines und Vergleichendes. In: Bethe, Bergmann, Embden-Ellinger, Handbuch der normalen und pathologischen Physiologie, Bd. 2, S. 1–36. Berlin: Springer 1925.

Biggs, P. M., King, A. S.: A new experimental approach to the problem of the air pathway within the avian lung. J. Physiol. (Lond.) 138, 282–289 (1957).

Brandes, G.: Atmung der Vögel. Verh. dtsch. zool. Ges. 28, 57–59 (1923).

— Beobachtungen und Reflexionen über die Atmung der Vögel. Pflügers Arch. ges. Physiol. 203, 492–511 (1924).

Breitenbach, R. P., Baskett, T. S.: Ontogeny of thermoregulation in the mourning dove. Physiol. Zool. 40, 207–217 (1967).

Bremer, J. L.: Evidence of an epithelial lining in the labyrinth of the avian lung. Anat. Rec. 73, 497–513 (1939).

Buddenbrock, W. v.: Atemmechanik der Vögel. In: Buddenbrock, Grundriß der vergleichenden Physiologie, S. 350–353. Berlin: Gebr. Borntraeger 1928.

Burkart, F., Bucher, K.: Elektromyographische Untersuchungen an der Atemmuskulatur der Taube. Helv. physiol. pharmacol. Acta 19, 263–268 (1961).

Burnstock, G.: Evolution of the autonomic innervation of visceral and cardiovascular systems in vertebrates. Pharmacol. Rev. 21, 247–324 (1969).

Butler, G. W.: Subdivision of body-cavity in lizards, crocodiles and birds. Proc. Zool. Soc. Lond. 1889, 452–474.

Calder, W. A.: Respiratory and heart rates of birds at rest. Condor 70, 358–365 (1968).

— Schmidt-Nielsen, K.: Temperature regulation and evaporation in the pigeon and the roadrunner. Amer. J. Physiol. 213, 883–889 (1967).

— — Panting and blood carbon dioxide in birds. Amer. J. Physiol. 215, 477–482 (1968).

Campana: Recherches d'anatomie, de physiologie et d'organogénie pour la détermination des lois de la genèse et de l'évolution des espèces animales. I. mémoire: Physiologie de la respiration chez les oiseaux, anatomie de l'appareil pneumatique-pulmonaire, des faux diaphragmes, des séreuses et de l'intestin chez le poulet. Paris: Masson 1875.

Camper, P.: Verhandeling over het zamenstel der groote Beenderen in Vogelen, en derzelven verscheidenheid in bijzondere soorten. Verh. van het Genootsch., Rotterdam 1774, 235–244, cit. according to Fischer 1905.

— Mémoire sur la structure des os dans les oiseaux et de leurs diversités dans les différentes espèces. Mém. math. phys. Acad. Sci. Paris 7, 328–335 (1776).

Chiodi, H., Terman, J. W.: Arterial blood gases of the domestic hen. Amer. J. Physiol. 208, 798–800 (1965).

Clements, J. A., Nellenbogen, J., Trahan, H. J.: Pulmonary surfactant and evolution of the lungs. Science 169, 603–605 (1970).

Cohn, J. E., Krog, J., Shannon, R.: Cardiopulmonary responses to head immersion in domestic geese. J. appl. Physiol. 25, 36–41 (1968).

— Shannon, R.: Respiration in unanesthetized geese. Resp. Physiol. 5, 259–268 (1968).

Coiter, V.: Anatomia Avium. In: Coiter, Externarum et internarum praecipalium humani corporis partium tabulae atque anatomicae exercitationes observationesque variae . . ., Norimbergae 1573, 130–133.

Colas: Essai sur l'organisation du poumon des oiseaux. J. complém. Dict. med., A. 23, 97–108 and 289–302 (1825), cit. to Campana 1875.

Comroe, J. H., Jr.: Physiologie der Atmung. Transl. by H. A. Gerlach and H. Bodenstab. Stuttgart-New York: Schattauer 1968.

Cook, R. D., King, A. S.: Nerves of the avian lung: electron microscopy. J. Anat. (Lond.) 105, 202–203 (1969a).

— — A neurite-receptor complex in the avian lung: Electron microscopical observations. Experientia (Basel) 25, 1162–1164 (1969b).

— — Observations on the ultrastructure of the smooth muscle and its innervation in the avian lung. J. Anat. (Lond.) 106, 273–284 (1970).

Cover, M. S.: Gross and microscopic anatomy of the respiratory system of the turkey. II. The larynx, trachea, syrinx, bronchi and lungs. Amer. J. vet. Res. 14, 230–238 (1953a).

— Gross and microscopic anatomy of the respiratory system of the turkey. III. The air sacs. Amer. J. vet. Res. 14, 239–245 (1953b).

Cowie, A. F., King, A. S.: Further observations on the bronchial muscle of birds. J. Anat. (Lond.) **104**, 177–178 (1969).

Crawford, E. C., Jr., Schmidt-Nielsen, K.: Temperature regulation and evaporative cooling in the ostrich. Amer. J. Physiol. **212**, 347–354 (1967).

Cuvier, G.: Vorlesungen über vergleichende Anatomie, gesammelt von G. L. Düvernoy und übersetzt von J. F. Meckel, Bd. 4. Leipzig: Kummer 1810.

Daniel, J. D., Jr.: An embryological comparison of the domestic fowl and the redwinged blackbird. Auk **74**, 340–358 (1957).

Dehner, E.: An apparatus for determining the respiratory volume of large aquatic birds. Science **103**, 171–172 (1946).

Delphia, J. M.: The origin of the air sacs in the white Pekin duck, *Anas platyrhynchos* L. Proc. North Dakota Acad. Sci. **12**, 86–92 (1958).

— Early development of the secondary bronchi in the house sparrow, *Passer domesticus* (L.). Amer. Midld Naturalist **65**, 44–59 (1961).

De Groodt, M., Sebruyns, M., Lagasse, A.: De ultra struktuur van de bloed-lucht-barriere in de long van vogels. Vlaams diergeneesk. T. **29**, 313–317 (1960).

De Wet, P. D., Fedde, M. R., Kitchell, R. L.: Innervation of the respiratory muscles of *Gallus domesticus*. J. Morph. **123**, 17–34 (1967).

Diesselhorst, G.: Klasse Aves, Vögel. In: Bertalanffy-Gessner, Handbuch der Biologie, Bd. VI, S. 745–866. Konstanz: Akad. Verlagsges. Athenaion Dr. Hachfeld 1964.

Dotterweich, H.: Versuche über den Weg der Atemluft in der Vogellunge. Z. vergl. Physiol. **11**, 271–284 (1930a).

— Die Bahnhofstauben und die Frage nach dem Weg der Atemluft. Zool. Anz. **90**, 253–262 (1930b).

— Ein weiterer Beitrag zur Atmungsphysiologie der Vögel. Z. vergl. Physiol. **18**, 803–809 (1933).

— Die Atmung der Vögel. Z. vergl. Physiol. **23**, 744–770 (1936).

Duncker, H.-R.: Der Bronchialbaum der Vogellunge. 62. Verh. Anat. Ges. Marburg 1967, Erg.-H. zu Anat. Anz. **121**, 287–292 (1968a).

— Der Lungenbau der Vögel und ihre Luftsäcke. 62. Verh. Anat. Ges. Marburg 1967, Erg.-H. zu Anat. Anz. **121**, 597–598 (1968b).

— Bautypen der Parabronchien der Vogellunge. 63. Verh. Anat. Ges. Leipzig 1968, Erg.-H. zu Anat. Anz. **125**, 297–302 (1969).

— Die Vogellunge — Palaeo- und Neopulmo. 64. Verh. Anat. Ges. Homburg/Saar 1969, Erg.-H. zu Anat. Anz. **126**, 491–496 (1970a).

— Die präparative Darstellung des Lungen-Luftsacksystems der Vögel. II. Tag. f. med.-morph. Präp.-Technik Rostock 1969. W. Z. Univ. Rostock **19**, 205–215 (1970b).

— Die Austauschoberfläche der Vogellunge — Quantitative Untersuchungen. 65. Verh. Anat. Ges. Würzburg 1970, Erg.-H. zu Anat. Anz. **128**, 373–375 (1971).

— Haufe, E., Schlüter, O.: Die Darstellung der Lungen und Luftsäcke der Vögel. I. Präparator **10**, 9–16 (1964).

— Schlüter, O.: Die Darstellung der Lungen und Luftsäcke der Vögel. II. Präparator **10**, 49–60 (1964).

Eberth, C. J.: Über den feineren Bau der Lunge. Z. wiss. Zool. **12**, 427–454 (1863).

Ede, D. A.: Bird structure. London: Hutchinson 1964.

Fabricius ab Aquapendente, H.: De respiratione et eius instrumentis. Padua 1615. (In: Fabricius, Opera omnia anatomiae et physiologicae. J. Kerckhem, Lugd. Batav. 1738, 161–186.)

Fedde, M. R.: Peripheral control of avian respiration. Fed. Proc. **29**, 1664–1673 (1970).

— Burger, R. E.: Death and pulmonary alterations following bilateral cervical vagotomy in the fowl. Poultry Sci. **42**, 1236–1246 (1963).

— — Kitchell, R. L.: The effect of anesthesia and age on respiration following bilateral, cervical vagotomy in the fowl. Poultry Sci. **42**, 1212–1223 (1963a).

— — — Localization of vagal afferents involved in the maintenance of normal avian respiration. Poultry Sci. **42**, 1224–1236 (1963b).

— — — Electromyographic studies of the effects of bodily position and anesthesia on the activity of the respiratory muscles of the domestic cock. Poultry Sci. **43**, 839–846 (1964a).

Fedde, M. R., Burger, R. E., Kitchell, R. L.: Electromyographic studies of the effects of bilateral, cervical vagotomy on the action of the respiratory muscles of the domestic cock. Poultry Sci. **43**, 1119–1125 (1964b).

— — — Anatomic and electromyographic studies of the costopulmonary muscles in the cock. Poultry Sci. **43**, 1177–1184 (1964c).

— Peterson, D. F.: Intrapulmonary receptor response to changes in airway-gas composition in *Gallus domesticus*. J. Physiol. (Lond.) **209**, 609–626 (1970).

Fischer, G.: Vergleichende anatomische Untersuchungen über den Bronchialbaum der Vögel. Zoologica **19**, H. 45, 1–46 (1905).

Fisher, H. J.: Avian anatomy 1925–1950, and some suggested problems. In: Wolfson, Recent studies in avian biology, p. 57–104. Urbana: Univ. Ill. Press 1955.

Fraenkel, G.: Der Atmungsmechanismus der Vögel während des Fluges. Biol. Zbl. **54**, 96–101 (1934).

Francois-Franck, M.: Etudes graphiques, photographiques de mécanique respiratoire comparée. C. R. Soc. Biol. (Paris) **58**/2, 174–176 (1906).

Frech, W.-E., Schultehinrichs, D., Vogel, H. R., Thews, G.: Modelluntersuchungen zum Austausch der Atemgase. I. Die O_2-Aufnahmezeiten des Erythrocyten unter den Bedingungen des Lungencapillarblutes. Pflügers Arch. ges. Physiol. **301**, 292–301 (1968).

Fürbringer, M.: Untersuchungen zur Morphologie und Systematik der Vögel, zugleich ein Beitrag zur Anatomie der Stütz- und Bewegungsorgane. I. Specieller Teil, Brust, Schulter und proximale Flügelregion der Vögel. Amsterdam: Van Holkema 1888.

— Zur vergleichenden Anatomie des Brustschulterapparates und der Schultermuskeln. Jena. Z. Med. Naturw. **36**, 289–736 (1902).

Fujiwara, T., Adams, F. H., Nozaki, M., Dermer, G. B.: Pulmonary surfactant phospholipids from turkey lung: comparison with rabbit lung. Amer. J. Physiol. **218**, 218–225 (1970).

Fuld, L.: De organis quibus aves spiritum ducunt. Diss. inaug., Wirceburgi 1816, cit. according to Retzius 1832, Campana 1875.

Gadow, H.: Vögel. I. Anatomischer Teil. In: Bronn's Klassen und Ordnungen des Thier-Reichs, Bd. 6, IV. Abt. Leipzig: Winter'sche Verlagsbuchhandlung 1891.

Gegenbaur, C.: Vergleichende Anatomie der Wirbelthiere mit Berücksichtigung der Wirbellosen, Bd. 2. Leipzig: Engelmann 1901.

Geoffroy-Saint-Hilaire, E.: Des organes respiratoires sous le rapport de la détermination et de l'identité de leurs pieces osseuses. In: Geoffroy-Saint-Hilaire, Philosophie anatomique, t. 1. Paris: Bailliere 1818.

George, J. C., Berger, A. J.: Avian myology. New York-London: Academic Press 1966.

Gerhartz, H.: Biochemie des Wachstums. Vergleich der chemischen Zusammensetzung einiger Organismen verschiedener Entwicklungsstufen. In: Junk, Oppenheimer und Pincussen, Tabulae Biologicae, Bd. 3, S. 581–589. Berlin: W. Junk 1926.

Gier, H. T.: The air sacs of the loon. Auk **69**, 40–49 (1952).

Gilbert, P. W.: The avian lung and air-sac system. Auk **56**, 57–63 (1939).

Gilliard, E. T., Steinbacher, G.: Vögel. In: Knaurs Tierreich in Farben. München-Zürich: Droemersche Verlagsanstalt 1959.

Goodrich, E. S.: Studies on the structure and development of vertebrates, vol. II. New York-London: Dover Publ. 1958.

Graham, J. D. P.: The air stream in the lung of the fowl. J. Physiol. (Lond.) **97**, 133–137 (1939).

Grau, H.: Die Respirationsorgane. In: Ellenberger-Baum, Handbuch der vergleichenden Anatomie der Haustiere, Anatomie der Hausvögel, S. 1095–1103. Berlin: Springer 1943.

Greenewalt, C. H.: Dimensional relationships for flying animals. Smithson. Misc. Coll. **144**, 1–46 (1962).

Groebbels, F.: Der Vogel. Bau, Funktion, Lebenserscheinung, Einpassung, Bd. 1, Atmungswelt und Nahrungswelt. Berlin: Gebr. Borntraeger 1932.

Grzimek, B., Meise, W., Niethammer, G., Steinbacher, J.: Vögel 2, Grzimeks Tierleben, Bd. 8. Zürich: Kindler 1969.

— — — Vögel 3, Grzimeks Tierleben, Bd. 9. Zürich: Kindler 1970.

— — — — Thenius, E.: Vögel 1, Grzimeks Tierleben, Bd. 7. Zürich: Kindler 1968.

Hart, J. S., Roy, O. Z.: Temperature regulation during flight in pigeons. Amer. J. Physiol. **213**, 1295–1298 (1967).

Harveus, G.: Exercitationes de generatione animalium. London 1651.

Hauge, A.: Hypoxia and pulmonary vascular resistance. The relative effects of pulmonary arterial and alveolar P_{O_2}. Acta physiol. scand. **76**, 121–130 (1969).

Hazelhoff, E. H.: Bouw en functie van de vogellong. Verslag van de gewonne vergaderingen der Afdeeling Natuurkunde, Amsterdam **52**, 391–400 (1943).

— Structure and function of the lung of birds. Poultry Sci. **30**, 3–10 (1951).

Herzog, K.: Anatomie und Flugbiologie der Vögel. Stuttgart: Fischer 1968.

Hunter, J.: An account of certain receptacles of air in birds which communicate with the lungs and are lodged both among the fleshy parts and in hollow bones of those animals. Phil. Trans. B **64**, 205–213 (1774) cit. according to Fischer 1905.

Huxley, T. H.: On the respiratory organs of *Apteryx*. Proc. Zool. Soc. Lond. 1882, 560–569.

Jones, D. R.: Avian afferent vagal activity related to respiratory and cardiac cycles. Comp. Biochem. Physiol. **28**, 961–966 (1969).

Juillet, A.: Observations comparatives sur les rapports du poumon et des sacs aériens chez les oiseaux. C. R. Acad. Sci. (Paris) **152**, 1330–1332 (1911a).

— Phases avancées du développement du poumon chez le poulet. C. R. Soc. Biol. (Paris) **70**, 985–986 (1911b).

— Rapports des sacs aériens et des bronches chez les oiseaux. C. R. Acad. Sci. (Paris) **152**, 1024–1026 (1911c).

— Recherches anatomiques embryologiques, histologiques et comparatives sur le poumon des oiseaux. Arch. Zool. exp. gén., sér. 5, **9**, 207–371 (1912a).

— A propos des bronches récurrentes du poumon des oiseaux. Arch. Zool. exp. gén., sér. 5, **10**, 26–28 (1912b).

Kayser, C.: Contribution à l'étude de la régulation thermique. L'émission d'eau et le rapport $H_2O : O_2$ chez quelques espèces homéothermes adultes et en cours de croissance. Ann. physiol. physiochim. biol. **6**, 721–744 (1930).

Kendeigh, S. C.: Effect of air temperature on the rate of energy metabolism in the English sparrow. J. exp. Zool. **96**, 1–16 (1944).

King, A. S.: The structure and function of the respiratory pathways of *Gallus domesticus*. Vet. Rec. **68**, 544–547 (1956).

— The aerated bones of *Gallus domesticus*. Acta anat. (Basel) **31**, 220–230 (1957).

— Structural and functional aspects of the avian lungs and airsacs. Int. Rev. Gen. Exp. Zool. **2**, 171–267 (1966).

— Atherton, J. D.: The identity of the air sacs of the turkey (*Meleagris gallopavo*). Acta anat. (Basel) **77**, 78–91 (1970).

— Cowie, A. F.: On the bronchial muscle of birds. J. Anat. (Lond.) **102**, 576 (1968).

— — The functional anatomy of the bronchial muscle of the bird. J. Anat. (Lond.) **105**, 323–336 (1969).

— Ellis, R. N. W., Watts, S. M. S.: Elastic fibres in avian lung. J. Anat. (Lond.) **101**, 607 (1967).

— McLelland, J., Molony, V., Bowsher, D., Mortimer, M., White, S. S.: On vagal afferent control of avian breathing. J. Anat. (Lond.) **104**, 182 (1969).

— — — Mortimer, M. F.: Respiratory afferent activity in the avian vagus: eupnoea, inflation and deflation. J. Physiol. (Lond.) **201**, 35P–36P (1969).

— Molony, V., McLelland, J., Bowsher, D. R., Mortimer, M. F.: Afferent respiratory pathways in the avian vagus. Experientia (Basel) **24**, 1017–1018 (1968).

— Payne, D. C.: The volumes of the lungs and air sacs in *Gallus domesticus*. J. Anat. (Lond.) **92**, 656 (1958).

— — The maximum capacities of the lungs and air sacs of *Gallus domesticus*. J. Anat. (Lond.) **96**, 495–503 (1962).

— — Normal breathing and the effects of posture in *Gallus domesticus*. J. Physiol. (Lond.) **174**, 340–347 (1964).

Krause, R.: Mikroskopische Anatomie der Wirbeltiere in Einzeldarstellungen. II. Vögel und Reptilien. Berlin-Leipzig: De Gruyter & Co. 1922.

Lack, D.: The height of bird migration. Brit. Birds **53**, 5–10 (1960).

Lambson, R. O., Cohn, J. E.: Ultrastructure of the lung of the goose and its lining of surface material. Amer. J. Anat. **122**, 631–649 (1968).

Larsell, O.: The development of recurrent bronchi and of air-sacs of the lung of the chick. Anat. Anz. **47**, 481–496 (1914).

Lasiewski, R. C., Dawson, W. R.: A re-examination of the relation between standard metabolic rate and body weight in birds. Condor **69**, 13–23 (1967).

— Weathers, W. W., Bernstein, M. H.: Physiological responses of the giant hummingbird *Patagona gigas*. Comp. Biochem. Physiol. **23**, 797–814 (1967).

Lehmann, G.: Kreislauf. In: Junk, Oppenheimer und Pincussen, Tabulae Biologicae, Bd. 1. Berlin: Junk 1925.

Lloyd, T. C., Jr.: Role of nerve pathways in the hypoxic vasoconstriction of lung. J. appl. Physiol. **21**, 1351–1355 (1966).

— Hypoxic pulmonary vasoconstriction: role of perivascular tissue. J. appl. Physiol. **25**, 560–565 (1968).

Locy, W. A., Larsell, O.: The embryology of the birds lungs. Based on observations of the domestic fowl. Part I. 1. The external aspects of lung development. 2. The development of the bronchial tree. Amer. J. Anat. **19**, 447–504 (1916a).

— — The embryology of the birds lungs. Based on observations of the domestic fowl. Part II. 3. The air sacs and the recurrent bronchi. Amer. J. Anat. **20**, 1–44 (1916b).

Lord, R. D., Jr., Bellrose, F. C., Cochran, W. W.: Radiotelemetry of the respiration of a flying duck. Science **137**, 39–40 (1962).

MacDonald, J. W.: Observations on the histology of the lung of *Gallus domesticus*. Brit. vet. J. **126**, 89–93 (1970).

MacMillen, R. E., Trost, C. H.: Thermoregulation and water loss in the Inca dove. Comp. Biochem. Physiol. **20**, 263–274 (1967).

Makowski, J.: Beitrag zur Klärung des Atmungsmechanismus der Vögel. Pflügers Arch. ges. Physiol. **240**, 407–418 (1938a).

— Beitrag zur Erklärung des Atemmechanismus bei Vögeln auf Grund von anatomischen, histologischen und physiologischen Untersuchungen. Kosmos (Łwówie) **63**, 87–120 (1938b).

Marcus, H.: Lungenstudie. V. Vergleichende Untersuchungen über die respiratorische Oberfläche und ihr Verhältnis zum Körpergewicht. Gegenbaurs morph. Jb. **59**, 561–566 (1928).

— Lungen. In:Bolk-Göppert-Kallius-Lubosch, Handbuch der vergleichenden Anatomie der Wirbeltiere, Bd. 3, S. 909–988. Berlin-Wien: Urban & Schwarzenberg 1937.

McLelland, J.: Observations with the light microscope on the ganglia and nerve plexuses of the intrapulmonary bronchi of the bird. J. Anat. (Lond.) **105**, 202 (1969).

Mennega, A., Calhoun, M. L.: Morphology of the lower respiratory structures of the white Pekin duck. Poultry Sci. **47**, 266–280 (1968).

Milne-Edwards, A.: Observations sur l'appareil respiratoire de quelques oiseaux. Ann. Sci. Nat. Zool., sér. V, **3**, 137–142 (1865).

Morgan, V. E., Chichester, D. F.: Properties of the blood of the domestic fowl. J. biol. Chem. **110**, 285–298 (1935).

Müller, B.: The air sacs of the pigeon. Smithson. Misc. Coll. **50**, 365–414 (1908).

Niethammer, G., Bauer, K. M., Glutz von Blotzheim, U. N.: Handbuch der Vögel Mitteleuropas, Bd. 1, *Gaviiformes-Phoenicopteriformes*. Frankfurt a.M.: Akad. Verlagsges. 1966.

— — — Handbuch der Vögel Mitteleuropas, Bd. 2, *Anseriformes* (1. Teil). Frankfurt a.M.: Akad. Verlagsges. 1968.

— — — Handbuch der Vögel Mitteleuropas, Bd. 3, *Anseriformes* (2. Teil). Frankfurt a.M.: Akad. Verlagsges. 1969.

Nisbet, J. C. T.: Measurements with radar of the height of nocturnal migration over Cape Cod, Massachusetts. Bird Banding **34**, 57–67 (1963).

— Drury, W. H., Jr., Baird, J.: Weight loss during migration. I. Deposition and consumption of fat by the blackpoll warbler *Dendroica striata*. Bird Banding **34**, 107–138 (1963).

Olander, H. J., Burton, R. R., Adler, H. E.: The pathophysiology of chronic hypoxia in chickens. Avian Diseases **11**, 609–620 (1967).

Oppel, A.: Atmungsapparat. In: Oppel, Lehrbuch der vergleichenden mikroskopischen Anatomie der Wirbeltiere, Bd. 6. Jena: Fischer 1905.

Owen, R.: On the anatomy of the gannet (*Sula bassana*). Proc. Zool. Soc. Lond. 1830, 90–92.
— Notes on the anatomy of the red-backed pelican (*Pelecanus rufescens*, Gmel.). Proc. Zool. Soc. Lond. 1835 a, 9–12.
— On the anatomy of the concave hornbill, *Buceros cavatus*. Transact. Zool. Soc. Lond. 1, 117–122 (1835 b).
— Respiratory system of birds. In: Owen, On the anatomy of vertebrates, vol. II: Birds and mammals, p. 205–225. London: Longmans, Green & Co. 1866.
Parker, W. N.: Note on the respiratory organs of *Rhea*. Proc. Zool. Soc. Lond. 1888, 141–142.
Pattle, R. E.: Properties, function and origin of the alveolar lining layer. Proc. roy. Soc. B 148, 217 (1958).
— The lining layer of the lung alveoli. Brit. med. Bull. 19, 41–44 (1963).
— Surface lining of lung alveoli. Physiol. Rev. 45, 48–79 (1965).
— Hopkinson, D. A. W.: Lung lining in bird, reptile and amphibian. Nature (Lond.) 200, 894 (1963).
Perrault, C.: Description anatomique de huit Autruches. Mem. hist. nat. anim. 1676, 167–181, cit. according to Campana 1875.
Peterson, D. F., Fedde, M. R.: Receptors sensitive to carbon dioxide in lungs of chicken. Science 162, 1499–1501 (1968).
Peterson, R., Mountfort, G., Hollom, P. A. D., Niethammer, G.: Die Vögel Europas, 6. Aufl. Hamburg-Berlin: Parey 1965.
Petrik, P.: The ultrastructure of the chicken lung in the final stages of embryonic development. Folia morph. (Prag) 15, 176–186 (1967).
— Riedel, B.: An osmiophilic bilaminar lining film at the respiratory surface of avian lungs. Z. Zellforsch. 88, 204–219 (1968 b).
— — A continuous osmiophilic noncellular membrane at the respiratory surface of the lungs of fetal chickens and of young chicks. Lab. Invest. 18, 54–62 (1968 a).
Petry, G.: Über die Formen und die Verteilungen elastisch-muskulöser Verbindungen in der Haut der Haustaube. Gegenbaurs morph. Jb. 91, 511–535 (1951).
Piiper, J., Drees, F., Scheid, P.: Gas exchange in the domestic fowl during spontaneous breathing and artificial ventilation. Resp. Physiol. 9, 234–245 (1970).
— Pfeifer, K., Scheid, P.: Carbon monoxide diffusing capacity of the respiratory system in the domestic fowl. Resp. Physiol. 6, 309–317 (1969).
Plantefol, A., Scharnke, H.: Contribution à l'étude du rôle des sacs aériens dans la respiration des oiseaux. Ann. Physiol. Physicochim. biol. 10, 83–85 (1934).
Policard, A., Collet, A., Martin, J. C.: La surface d'échange air-sang dans le poumon oiseaux. Etude au microscope électronique. Z. Zellforsch. 57, 37–46 (1962).
Poole, M.: The development of the subdivisions of the pleuroperitoneal cavity in birds. Proc. Zool. Soc. Lond. 49, 210–235 (1909).
Portier, P.: Sur le rôle physiologique des sacs aériens des oiseaux. C. R. Soc. Biol. (Paris) 99, 1327–1328 (1928).
Portmann, A.: Les organes de la circulation sanguine. In: Grassé, Traité de Zoologie, t. XV, Oiseaux, p. 243–256. Paris: Masson 1950 a.
— Les organes respiratoires. In: Grassé, Traité de Zoologie, t. XV, Oiseaux, p. 257–269. Paris: Masson 1950 b.
Rainey, G.: On the minute anatomy of the lung of the bird, considered chiefly in relation to the structure with which the air is in contact whilst traversing the ultimate subdivisions of the air passages. Med.-chir. Trans. 32, 47–58 (1849).
Rathke, H.: Über die Entwicklung der Athmungswerkzeuge bei den Vögeln und Säugethieren. Nov. Act. Acad. Leop. Carol. 14, 159–216 (1828).
Ray, P. J., Fedde, M. R.: Responses to alterations in respiratory P_{O_2} and P_{CO_2} in the chicken. Resp. Physiol. 6, 135–143 (1969).
Remane, A.: Wirbelsäule und ihre Abkömmlinge. In: Bolk-Göppert-Kallius-Lubosch, Handbuch der vergleichenden Anatomie der Wirbeltiere, Bd. 4, S. 1–206. Berlin-Wien: Urban & Schwarzenberg 1936.
Retzius, A.: Einige Worte über den wahren Bau der Vögel-Lungen. Froriep's Notiz. 35, 1–9 (1832).

Richards, S. A.: Vagal function during respiration and the effects of vagotomy in the domestic fowl (Gallus domesticus). Comp. Biol. Physiol. 29, 955–964 (1969).

Richardson, F.: Functional aspects of the pneumatic system of the California Brown Pelican. Condor 41, 13–17 (1939).

Rigdon, R. H.: The respiratory system in the normal white Pekin duck. Poultry Sci. 38, 196–210 (1959).

Roche, G.: Contribution à l'étude de l'anatomie comparée des réservoirs aériens d'origine pulmonaires chez les oiseaux. Ann. Sci. Nat., Sér. VII, Zool. 11, 1–120 (1891).

Romanoff, A. L.: The avian embryo. New York: Macmillan & Co. 1960.

Romeis, B.: Mikroskopische Technik, 15. Aufl. München: Leibniz Verlag 1948.

Saalfeld, E. von: Untersuchungen über das Hacheln bei Tauben. Z. vergl. Physiol. 23, 727–743 (1936).

Salt, G. W.: Respiratory evaporation in birds. Biol. Rev. 39, 113–136 (1964).

— Zeuthen, E.: The respiratory system. In: Marshall, Biology and comparative physiology of birds, vol. 1, p. 363–409. New York-London: Academic Press 1960.

Sappey, P. C.: Recherches sur l'appareil respiratoire des oiseaux. Paris: Germer-Bailliere 1847.

Scarpelli, E. M.: Surfactant system of the lung. Philadelphia: Lea & Febiger 1968.

Scharnke, H.: Die Bedeutung der Luftsäcke für die Atmung der Vögel. Ergebn. Biol. 10, 177–206 (1934).

— Experimentelle Beiträge zur Kenntnis der Vogelatmung. Z. vergl. Physiol. 25, 548–583 (1938).

Scheid, P., Piiper, J.: Messung einiger atemphysiologischer Größen am Huhn. Pflügers Arch. ges. Physiol. 297, R46 (1967).

— — Messungen zum Gasaustausch am Huhn: Vergleich mit einem Modell der Vogellunge. Pflügers Arch. ges. Physiol. 300, 17 (1968).

— — Volume, ventilation and compliance of the respiratory tract in the domestic fowl. Resp. Physiol. 6, 298–308 (1969).

— — Analysis of gas exchange in the avian lung: Theory and experiments in the domestic fowl. Resp. Physiol. 9, 246–262 (1970).

— — Direct measurement of the pathway of respired gas in duck lungs. Resp. Physiol. 11, 308–314 (1971).

Schoedel, W., Rüfer, R.: Veränderungen der Oberflächenverhältnisse in den Lungenalveolen als Ursache von Atelektasen und gestörter Atemmechanik. Dtsch. med. Wschr. 93, 1623–1628 (1968).

Scholander, P. F.: Experimental investigation on the respiratory function in diving mammals and birds. Hvalråd Skrifter Oslo 22, 1–131 (1940).

Schmidt-Nielsen, K., Hainsworth, F. R., Murrish, D. E.: Countercurrent heat exchange in the respiratory passages: effect on water and heat balance. Resp. Physiol. 9, 263–276 (1970).

Schulze, F. E.: Die Lungen der Vögel. In: Stricker, Handbuch der Lehre von den Geweben der Menschen und der Thiere, Bd. 1, S. 477–480. Leipzig: Engelmann 1871.

— Die Lungen des afrikanisches Straußes. S.-B. preuß. Akad. Wiss., Berlin 1908, 416–431.

— Über die Funktion der Luftsäcke bei den Vögeln. S.-B. preuß. Akad. Wiss., Berlin 1909, 631.

— Über die Bronchi saccales und den Mechanismus der Atmung bei den Vögeln. S.-B. preuß. Akad. Wiss., Berlin 1910, 537–538.

— Über die Luftsäcke der Vögel, Verh. 8. Int. Zool.-Kongr., Graz 1910, S. 446–482. Jena: Fischer 1912.

Scott, P., Klös, H.-G.: Das Wassergeflügel der Welt. Hamburg-Berlin: Parey 1961.

Seeliger, H.: Quantitative Untersuchungen an Albinomäusen (erbreiner Stamm „Agnes Bluhm"). Absolute und relative Gewichte von Gehirn, Herz, Lunge, Leber, Milz, Nieren und Hoden. Anat. Anz. 109, 51–73 (1960).

Selenka, E.: Beitrag zur Entwicklung der Luftsäcke des Huhnes. Z. wiss. Zool. 16, 178–182 (1866).

Shaw, J. W.: Direct evidence for a dilatator action of carbon dioxid in pulmonary vessels when vascular tone is high. J. Physiol. (Lond.) 207, 75P (1970).

Shepard, R. H., Sladen, B. K., Peterson, N. Enns T.: Path taken by gases through the respiratory system of the chicken. J. appl. Physiol. 14, 733–735 (1959).

Siefert, E.: Über die Athmung der Reptilien und Vögel. II. Hauptteil: Die Athmung der Vögel. Pflügers Arch. ges. Physiol. 64, 428–506 (1896).

Simons, J. R.: The blood-vascular system. In: Marshall, Biology and comparative physiology of birds, vol. I, p. 345–362. New York-London: Academic Press 1960.

Soum, J. H.: Recherches physiologiques sur l'appareil respiratoire des oiseaux. Ann. l'université Lyon 28, 1–126 (1896).

Spells, K. E.: Some physical considerations relevant to the dimensions of lung alveoli. Nature (Lond.) 219, 64–66 (1968).

Stanislaus, M.: Untersuchungen an der Kolibrilunge. Z. Morph. Ökol. Tiere 33, 261–289 (1937).

— Böhme, W.: Röntgenkinematographische Studien über Vogelatmung. Zool. Anz., Suppl. 11, 179–182 (1938).

Stannius, H.: Lehrbuch der vergleichenden Anatomie der Wirbelthiere. Berlin: Veit & Co. 1846.

Steen, I., Steen, J. B.: The importance of the legs in the thermoregulation of birds. Acta physiol. scand. 63, 285–291 (1965).

Stolpe, M., Zimmer, K.: Atmungs- und Luftsacksystem, Luftzirkulation. In: Berndt-Meise, Naturgeschichte der Vögel, Bd. 1, Allgemeine Vogelkunde, S. 134–141. Stuttgart: Franckh'sche Verlagsbuchhandlung 1959.

Strasser, H.: Die Luftsäcke der Vögel. Gegenbaurs morph. Jb. 3, 179–225 (1877).

Stresemann, E.: Sauropsidae: Aves. In: Kükenthal-Krumbach, Handbuch der Zoologie, Bd. 7/2. Berlin-Leipzig: De Gruyter & Co. 1927–1934.

Sturkie, P. D.: Avian physiology, 2nd ed. New York: Comstock Publ. 1965.

Tenney, S. M., Remmers, J. E.: Comparative quantitative morphology of the mammalian lung: diffusing area. Nature (Lond.) 197, 54–56 (1963).

Thilo, O.: Die Luftsäcke der Vögel als Sperrvorrichtungen. Riga: W. F. Häcker 1915.

Tomlinson, J. T.: Breathing of birds in flight. Condor 65, 514–516 (1963).

— McKinnon, R. S.: Pigeon wing-beats synchronized with breathing. Condor 59, 401 (1957).

Tucker, V. A.: Respiratory exchange and evaporative water loss in the flying budgerigar. J. exp. Biol. 48, 67–88 (1968a).

— Respiratory physiology of house sparrows in relation to high-altitude flight. J. exp. Biol. 48, 55–66 (1968b).

— The energetics of bird flight. Sci. Amer. 220, 70–81 (1969).

Tyler, W. S., Pangborn, J.: Laminated membrane surface and osmiophilic inclusions in avian lung epithelium. J. Cell Biol. 20, 157–164 (1964).

Victorow, C.: Die kühlende Wirkung der Luftsäcke bei Vögeln. Pflügers Arch. ges. Physiol. 126, 300–322 (1909).

Vince, M. A., Salter, S. H.: Respiration and clicking in quail embryos. Nature (Lond.) 216, 582–583 (1967).

Visschedijk, A. H. J.: The air space and embryonic respiration. I. The pattern of gaseous exchange in the fertile egg during the closing stages of incubation. Brit. Poult. Sci. 9, 173–184 (1968a).

— The air space and embryonic respiration. II. The times of pipping and hatching as influenced by an artificially changed permeability of the shell over the air space. Brit. Poult. Sci. 9, 185–196 (1968b).

— The air space and embryonic respiration. III. The balance between oxygen and carbon dioxide in the air space of the incubating chicken egg and its role in stimulating pipping. Brit. Poult. Sci. 9, 197–210 (1968c).

Vos, H. J.: Über die Wege der Atemluft in der Entenlunge. Z. vergl. Physiol. 21, 552–578 (1935).

— Über das Fehlen der rekurrenten Bronchien beim Pinguin und bei den Reptilien. Zool. Anz. 117, 176–181 (1937).

Walter, W. G.: Beiträge zur Frage über den Weg der Luft in den Atmungsorganen der Vögel. Arch. neerl. Physiol. 19, 529–537 (1934).

Wastl, H., Leiner, G.: Beobachtungen über die Blutgase bei den Vögeln. I.–III. Pflügers Arch. ges. Physiol. **227**, 367–474 (1931).

Weber, E.: Bau der Lungen und Mechanismus des Athmens bei den Vögeln. 19. Verh. Ges. dtsch. Naturf. Ärzte, Braunschweig 1841, S. 75–78. Braunschweig: Vieweg & Sohn 1842.

Weibel, E. R.: Morphometry of the human lung. Berlin-Göttingen-Heidelberg: Springer 1963.

Wetherbee, D. K.: Airsacs in the English sparrow. Auk **68**, 242–244 (1951).

Wick, H., Bucher, K.: Charakteristika einer aktiven Exspiratorität bei der Taube. Helv. physiol. pharmacol. Acta **21**, 165–172 (1963).

Zeuthen, E.: The ventilation of the respiratory tract in birds. Kgl. danske Vid. Selsk. biol. Medd. 17, 1–51 (1942).

Zimmer, K.: Beiträge zur Mechanik der Atmung bei den Vögeln in Stand und Flug. Auf Grund anatomisch-physiologischer und experimenteller Studien. Zoologica **33**/5, Heft 88, 1–69 (1935).

Subject Index

Ergebnisse der Anatomie
und Entwicklungsgeschichte

Advances in Anatomy
Embryology and Cell Biology

Revues d'anatomie
et de morphologie expérimentale

Editores
A. Brodal, Oslo · W. Hild, Galveston · R. Ortmann, Köln
T. H. Schiebler, Würzburg · G. Töndury, Zürich · E. Wolff, Paris

Band 45 (Heft 1—6)

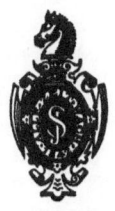

Springer-Verlag Berlin Heidelberg GmbH 1971

ISBN 978-3-540-05659-1   ISBN 978-3-662-10354-8 (eBook)
DOI 10.1007/978-3-662-10354-8

Inhalt / Contents